I00933687

The Challenge of Regulating Managed Care

Michigan Forum on Health Policy

Series Editor: Marilynn M. Rosenthal

The Challenge of Regulating Managed Care, by John E. Billi and
    Gail B. Agrawal, Editors

A Note from the Series Editor

This book, and the multimedia health policy series of which it is a part, is pred-
icated on a central belief: That social policy is best understood through the juxtaposition of positions, perspectives, ideas, and ideologies. These include the
political, organizational, institutional, social science, and historical. This naturally produces a clash of perspectives among the social scientist, the bureaucrat,
the policy maker, the politician, the practitioner, and the consumer.

Our central purpose is to lay out those different views, articulated by the
best people we can find. Of course the editors have their own biases and preferences. We have tried to put them aside and help our audience and readers
clarify and understand varying viewpoints. We are dedicated to raising standards for information and for judging "facts," sometimes pointing out how
difficult it is to establish " facts." Often, positions and ideologies are based on
assumptions, and sometimes issues are so complex that is the best we can do.

Presented first as a symposium at the University of Michigan, this book
reflects that commitment to juxtaposition. How else can we understand the
dynamic and confounding context within which we discuss and build social
policy in American democracy?

Join us in exploring the complexities of formulating, legislating, implementing, and evaluating health policy across a variety of current and pressing
national concerns.

University of Michigan FORUMS will appear in book, article, web site, and
journal supplement forms.

Watch www.med.umich.edu/psm/FORUM.html for details.

Marilynn M. Rosenthal, Ph.D.
Professor and Director, University of Michigan FORUM on Health Policy
Ann Arbor, Michigan

The Challenge of Regulating Managed Care

Edited by
John E. Billi
and
Gail B. Agrawal

Ann Arbor
THE UNIVERSITY OF MICHIGAN PRESS

2004   2003   2002   2001   4   3   2   1

A CIP catalog record for this book is available from the British Library.

Library of Congress Cataloging-in-Publication Data

The challenge of regulating managed care / edited by John E. Billi and
     Gail B. Agrawal.
        p. ; cm. — (Michigan forum on health policy)
     Includes bibliographical references and index.
     ISBN 0-472-09778-4 (cloth : alk. paper)
     1. Managed care plans (Medical care)
     [DNLM: 1. Managed Care Programs—organization &
     administration—United States.   2. Health Policy—United States. W
     130 AA1 C437 2001] I. Billi, John E.   II. Agrawal, Gail B. (Gail
     Bopp), 1951–   III. Title.   IV. Series.
     RA413 .C45   2001   2001002124

Contents

Acknowledgments

The editors gratefully acknowledge the contributions of the following people to the completion of this work. Thanks to series editor Marilynn M. Rosenthal for inviting us to undertake this interesting project and for shepherding us through the process; to our University of Michigan Press editors, Rebecca McDermott, Liz Suhay, and Ellen McCarthy; to Carol L. Kent for expert manuscript preparation and editorial assistance; and to Raj Gupta, University of Michigan Inteflex medical student, for preparing the extensive list of on-line resources found in Appendix B. A special thanks goes to Jeanne Kin for project coordination.

PART 1

Understanding the Big Picture

Managing the Managers: An Introduction to the Challenge of Overseeing Managed Care

Gail B. Agrawal

This monograph on the challenge of regulating the managed-care industry has its origins in a health policy forum held at the University of Michigan Medical School. The forum brought together a well-known journalist-author, leaders of organized medicine and the managed-care industry, consumer advocates, and health-care scholars on the faculty at the University of Michigan to discuss difficult issues related to managing health-care services and health-care costs. As my co-editor and I discussed the forum and the ideas raised there, we decided to include in this monograph additional viewpoints on the pressing social issues that surround the industry commonly called "managed care."[1] We invited other stakeholders, including representatives of large employers, the government, and academic medical centers, to share their views on the oversight of the managed-care industry. Within this book's pages, the reader will hear from economists, physicians, lawyers, business executives, lawmakers, and policy analysts on this complex subject.

Although the authors' diverse views are expressed in the context of managed care, they are a microcosm of the larger societal debate surrounding the inevitable trade-off among health-care quality, cost, and access in an environment of limited resources. The modern managed-care industry is merely the current manifestation of an ongoing effort to determine how and by whom that trade-off will be made. The authors' diverse opinions about the oversight of the managed-care industry also reflect the enduring perspectives of important stakeholders in the larger debate. As each author presents the view of a single stakeholder, the text that emerges is a serendipitously presented comparative institutional analysis that considers the effectiveness of legislation, judicial decision making, and competition in achieving an appropriate balance for health care.

My goal for this introductory chapter is modest and twofold. First, this chapter provides an overview of managed care and the evolving role of the legal system in its development and oversight. Second, it is intended both to frame the debate between proponents of legal regulation and of market oversight generally and to preview the specific views of the contributing authors on this debate in the managed-care context.

The Role of Law in the Evolution of Managed Care

The term *managed care* is used to describe a wide range of disparate benefit designs that combine health-care services and health-care coverage with the goal of reducing, or at least containing, health-care spending.[2] The present-day managed-care industry traces its origins to prepaid group practices established prior to World War I.[3] These group practices followed the railroads into the then remote region of the American Northwest.[4] Like modern-day managed care, early prepaid medical practice was employer based: physicians contracted with large employers to deliver health-care services to their employees for a fixed sum per employee per month. The Kaiser Permanente system is frequently cited as the earliest commercial managed-care plan. It began as a not-for-profit, prepaid plan to provide care to workers on construction projects in California and later to shipyard workers during World War II.[5] These pioneers in prepaid health care envisioned the delivery of affordable health-care services with a focus on preventive care to be provided in an outpatient setting. Their services were rendered primarily to underserved populations of patients in defined geographic regions. Most early enrollees in prepaid medical care plans were working men and women and their children. The elderly, the disabled, and the chronically ill were rare among early managed-care participants. In caring for the same patients over extended periods, physicians hoped to reduce the cost of care by interceding to maintain health and to prevent illnesses that required high-intensity medical services.

The managed-care industry has expanded well beyond this initial niche. It is no longer limited to underserved populations of working individuals and their families residing in remote areas. Managed care has become the coverage of choice for large and small employers in urban and suburban areas.[6] It is also making inroads into the elderly, the disabled, and the indigent population through contracts with the federal and state governments to provide care and coverage to Medicare and Medicaid beneficiaries. In addition, managed-care organizations no longer rely on a stable group of physicians to provide care to a constant group of patients. Increasingly, managed-care organizations enter annual contracts with large numbers of independent physicians and physician organizations whose practices are not limited to a single organization. These contracts give both payer and caregiver the option to terminate the relationship on relatively short notice. As managed-care organizations compete for the business of large group purchasers, the annual purchasing decision can affect the stability of a large number of patient-physician relationships.

Volatile stock prices and ever larger managed-care entities are more characteristic of modern-day perceptions of managed care than are idealistic physicians aspiring to provide health care at a reasonable cost to underserved populations. Today the managed-care industry offers corporate purchasers a wide range of health benefit designs, including health maintenance organizations, preferred provider organizations, exclusive provider options, and point-of-service (POS) plans. These coverage options are offered through a varied array of organizations, from large indemnity insurers to freestanding health maintenance organizations to self-insured employer plans. The most recent entrant into the marketplace is the provider-sponsored organization, which might take the form of a physician-controlled independent practice association, a hospital-physician entity joint venture, or an integrated delivery system. In stark contrast to the early participants in the managed-care arena, most entities now participating in the marketplace are organized as for-profit corporations, many of which are publicly traded.

The present-day managed-care industry has often been characterized as a marketplace response to the perceived need for health-care reform of a system based on fee for service medicine and indemnity insurance. In the traditional fee-for-service delivery system, physicians ordered, payers paid, and insured patients largely avoided the economic consequences of their health-care choices. The professional model for health-care delivery reigned, and physicians, not patients, made decisions about the services that would be provided and the quality of those services. These traits combined to cause unsustainable levels of health-care spending. Managed care, with cost control as a principal focus, was seen as a way out of the spiral.

Proponents of unfettered market forces as a means to oversee the managed-care industry sometimes rely on the characterization of managed care as market-driven reform to support their position that government regulation is at best unwarranted and at worse counterproductive to the goals of cost-effective quality health care. The characterization of managed care as a product of unfettered market forces created on a level playing field with other health-care delivery and financing systems, however, ignores at least some part of its history. Managed care in its current form, expanded well beyond construction and shipyard workers and their families, could be viewed as an offspring of federal legislation. The enforcement of federal antitrust laws to the so-called learned professions contributed significantly to the shift from a professional paradigm of health-care delivery to a market model of health-care delivery.[7] For purchasers and payers to influence health care the physician monopoly on medical care had to be moderated.

Federal legislation enacted in the 1970s both removed barriers and provided assistance to the fledgling managed-care industry. Mandatory health planning preceded the advent of managed care as the preferred legislative model for cost control in health care. It built upon the coordinated, collective activity among health-care professionals and health-care institutions that characterized the professional model for health-care delivery. In 1974 Congress enacted the National Health Planning and Resource Development Act (NHPRDA).[8] That statute required states to establish health planning oversight agencies to consider requests for substantial spending on health-care resources and to grant or deny certificates of need that were required by the legislation. Without a certificate of need, health-care institutions were not entitled to reimbursement under the Medicare or Medicaid programs. Some states went further than the federal law required and elected to prohibit entirely any major expenditure on health-care resources for which a certificate of need was denied.[9] In those states, hospitals could not expand, new nursing homes could not be constructed, and expensive pieces of diagnostic equipment could not be purchased without government authorization. Health maintenance organizations, however, were exempt from the NHPRDA and, thus, from the requirement that they receive a certificate of need to acquire new facilities or make major investments in health-care technology.[10] Congress protected health maintenance organizations from this law to foster their development, viewing the managed-care movement and market competition as an alternative means to mandated health planning to control health-care spending.

During this same period, Congress enacted the Health Maintenance Organization Act (HMO Act)[11] and the Employee Retirement Income Security Act,[12] statutes that are discussed throughout this monograph. The former provided start-up funds for federally qualified health maintenance organizations and protected them from state laws that would hamper their growth. The federal HMO Act also afforded federally qualified health maintenance organizations the ability to mandate their way into the marketplace for health-care coverage by enabling them to require that certain employers offer a managed-care option to their employees.[13] Within a decade after the enactment of the HMO Act, states followed the federal lead, enacting enabling legislation for health maintenance organizations.[14] The HMO Act gradually lost its importance as fewer health maintenance organizations elected to obtain federally qualified status, but not before it fostered significant growth in the managed-care sector.[15]

The federal legislation most protective of managed-care entities in effect, if not in original intent, was the Employee Retirement Income Security Act of 1974 (ERISA). As Peter D. Jacobson discusses in chapter 13, the most significant effect on health benefit plans has been ERISA's preemption of state laws that "related to" ERISA plans. By preempting state laws that related to ERISA plans, the federal law provided managed-care organizations that covered ERISA plan beneficiaries with a protective shield from liability under state common law doctrines and from direct state regulation for many of their cost containment activities. Although the impenetrability of the ERISA shield for managed-care organizations has begun to erode, this federal law has done much to enable managed-care organizations to develop cost containment strategies relatively unhampered by the fear of private lawsuits or burdensome state laws.

Thus began the role of the law in the modern-day reformation of the financing and delivery of health care in the United States. Federal law played a significant part in creating the playing field on which the market nurtured the growth of managed care. Over time, managed-care organizations came to dominate the health-care marketplace. Anecdotes of tragic results became commonplace. And the focus of the state and federal law shifted from encouraging the expansion of managed care to controlling the perceived excesses of the managed-care industry in its quest to control the cost of health-care services.

The principal question addressed in this monograph is whether the legal system has a continuing role to play in the oversight of managed care and, if so, what that role might be. An alternative question is whether the oversight of managed care should be entrusted largely, or even solely, to market forces.[16] Proponents of regulatory oversight point to failures or imperfections in the market for health-care services to justify their position that more regulation, not less, is necessary to protect consumers in the present and health-care delivery in the future. The lack of understandable information and meaningful choice and the ability to exit one competitor for another all militate against market oversight for health care. Market advocates counter that legislation too has its imperfections. It is subject to capture by organized medicine and other special interests groups, serving their interests rather than the needs of health-care consumers. They maintain that a free market will produce the right mix of third-party payers for health care services through consumer choice in the marketplace. Those favoring the market over legislation also contend that legislation both increases costs to group purchasers and consumers and impedes the ability of managed-care organizations to respond quickly to purchaser demand. Market forces, proponents argue, will eliminate managed-care practices that are not favored by consumers, making government intervention unnecessary.

Although managed-care benefit designs vary widely, most managed-care plans share common elements. Managed-care models are network-based benefit designs that include both negative and positive incentives to caregivers to control the cost of health care. Managed-care plans also exercise varying degrees of direct control of the delivery and cost of care. In planning for this monograph, we suggested to the authors that they consider these common aspects of managed care and address whether and how managed-care organizations might be held accountable for them.

An Overview

The monograph begins with George Anders's national overview of the public perception and government regulation of the managed-care industry. He answers the question of "regulation or market forces" with a resounding vote for regulation. Anders maintains that government regulation is necessary in managed care for two reasons. First, he asserts that the purchasing decision for health-care coverage—the demand side of the equation—is different than that for other market commodities. Insurance purchase decisions are made long before health-care needs are known. In addition, decisions about the use of health-care services are made at times of great anxiety and vulnerability. On the supply side, he points out, not all consumers of insurance are equally desirable to insurers. A market-based insurance system will never respond to the needs of those individuals or segments of the population whose requirements for health-care services make them inevitably unprofitable to insure. Anders urges consensus building among four interest groups—consumers, physicians, employers, and insurers—as a means to achieve responsible regulation of managed care. Appropriate regulation, he contends, will enable the industry to achieve its potential for cost control and coordinated care.

Drawing on his perspective as a journalist, Anders recounts the public backlash against managed care and the legislative initiatives that can be traced to public outrage over some managed-care practices. As examples he points to maternity length-of-stay laws enacted by many states and the federal government after some health maintenance organizations adopted guidelines that called for the discharge of mother and baby within twenty-four hours of a normal vaginal delivery and laws prohibiting so-called gag clauses (managed-care contract terms that restrict physicians' communication with their patients). In later chapters, other authors, notably Keith J. Crocker and John R. Moran, point to a study by the General Accounting Office that tends to prove that gag clauses were not in widespread use, despite the public outcry about them.

Professor Alice A. Noble and Dr. Troy A. Brennan put the legislation described by Anders into context by identifying temporal patterns of legislative activity. In stage 1, during the 1970s and 1980s, legislation promoted managed care. By the mid-1990s, we had entered into stage 2, which Noble and Brennan characterize as the anti-managed-care regulatory period. Laws enacted during this period were narrowly targeted and reflexive rather than part of a comprehensive regulatory strategy. They also highlight the influence of organized medicine's resistance to the shift from a caregiver-dominated fee-for-service model to a managed-care system. In stage 3, discernible patterns began to emerge, with copycat legislation among the states and a growing federal presence. Much of the legislation described in Anders's chapter falls into this period, as legislators attempted to respond to consumers' concerns about managed care. Noble and Brennan describe the current period as a "regulatory middle ground" between consumer backlash and market forces.

Like Anders, Noble and Brennan envision a regulatory environment for managed-care oversight. They propose establishing through federal legislation a floor for consumer protections that is based on societal consensus. They call for federal mandates for disclosures to enrollees, consumer choice of providers and plans, and consumer protection from onerous managed-care requirements such as access to specialists and emergency room care, among other patient protections. They also support legislation that would respond to perceived market imperfections in consumer information, requiring standardized reporting requirements and uniform disclosure of data. Their and Anders's reliance on societal consensus is a sharp contrast from market proponents' criticism of the democratic political process that appears in its starkest form in chapter 8 by Bruce Bradley and his coauthors writing for the industry giant General Motors (GM).

In Dr. Clifton R. Cleaveland's chapter, the reader moves from a dispassionate discussion of legislation and managed care to a description of managed care as seen from the perspectives of caregivers. Cleaveland writes as a leader of the American College of Physicians and as a longtime practicing physician. In his view, the current managed-care system is characterized by "chaos, consolidation, micromanagement, and unrestrained administrative misbehavior." He opines that the quality of care in a managed-care system "sinks to the lowest common denominator" due to the rigidity imposed by managed-care payment policies. He relies on physician surveys to report on large-scale dissatisfaction with managed care in clinical practice. The current system is also denounced for its failure to provide care and the protection of insurance for all citizens.

Cleaveland, running counter to payers' stereotypes of physicians, does not advocate a return to a fee-for-service system, a system he characterizes as fraught with "needless medical testing, administrative costs, insurance abuse, and fraud." Rather, he proposes a federal regulatory system that would ensure for all Americans a uniform, evidence-based package of health-care benefits. In this model, panels of physicians and public health experts would define the benefit package. He joins Noble and Brennan in suggesting that federal law should establish legal rights for patients, and he adds that the law should also provide rights for caregivers. The system he envisions would be a private managed-care insurance system funded by a mixture of private and public moneys. Addressing problems identified by Dr. John E. Billi and Jeanne M. Kin in their chapter about the academic medical center and managed care, Cleaveland proposes a system that would include an all-payer tax to support medical education and research. In a sharp break with the traditional notion of unfettered self-regulation as the sole valid model for professional oversight, Cleaveland states that the model he envisions would include federally appointed arbiters to resolve issues of clinical privileges for caregivers.

Chapter 5 provides the insights of another group that is personally and profoundly affected by the shift from fee-for-service medicine and indemnity insurance to a managed-care system. Cathy L. Hurwit writes of the patient-consumer perspective. She concurs with Cleaveland that the actual result of managed care has been a reduction in the quality of and access to care. Relying on different sources of data, she too reports on physician and patient dissatisfaction with managed care. While noting some studies that suggest that clinical outcomes are no worse in a managed-care system than they are in a fee-for-service indemnity system, she points to other studies that show that families in poor health rate managed care lower than indemnity plans.

Hurwit adds the consumers' voice to those reflected in previous chapters in calling for a legislative solution to the health-care dilemma. She contends that market forces will not result in a managed-care system that improves patient care and that is accountable for its actions. In her view, the specialized nature of health care means that reliance on informed consumers is misplaced, even if consumers were able to select their own insurers and coverage options. She maintains that additional information would not markedly improve the functioning of the market, because of the complexity of information required to make informed decisions and the individual needs of consumers. More important, however, she points to the failings of even a "perfect" market. Market forces will not ensure legal protections or provide a participatory role for consumers. She urges "comprehensive systemic reforms" to ensure rights for all health-care consumers regardless of health status, age, sex, race, or geographic location, with special attention to the needs of the chronically ill, senior citizens, low-income individuals, and persons with disabilities. Among these rights, she includes timely access to appropriate care, choice of qualified professionals and affordable comprehensive plans, a voice in health plan decision making, and the right to a fair process to challenge decisions about practices that affect access and quality.

The final chapter in this section on those who give and receive care in a managed-care system is by Dr. John Billi and Jeanne M. Kin, who describe the challenges presented by managed care for the academic medical center. Academic medical centers are an important part of any health-care delivery system. There the sickest and the poorest patients receive care; young physicians hone their skills and are trained in the art of medicine; and scientists conduct the research that will improve health and medical care in the future. As a result of these special missions, academic medical centers are expensive to operate and are high-cost providers of care. Managed care, with its emphasis on managing health-care costs, shuns academic medical centers even as they confront the task of educating young physicians for practice in a system dominated by managed care and population-based medicine.

Academic medical centers have responded to managed care in a number of ways. First, they strive to become more like their nonteaching institution counterparts to control costs. In this role, academic medical centers tend to share the views of other health-care institutions on the subject of managed-care regulation. They favor patient and provider protection. They are also, however, well placed to develop their own managed-care plans. When an academic medical center elects to own and operate its own managed-care plan, it begins to mirror the views of commercial managed-care plans that prefer competition to regulation.

The juxtaposition of the academic medical center both as a provider and as a managed-care plan competing in the marketplace brings the reader to the next section of the monograph. Part 3 opens with a chapter by Professors Keith J. Crocker and John R. Moran. They tackle an argument that is either made explicitly or implied in each of the previous chapters: medical care is unique, and, therefore, application of standard economic principles is inappropriate. Resorting to a device that I have discussed elsewhere,[17] they compare health insurance to car insurance and conclude that both suffer from information and incentive problems. Consumers of health care or car care are generally uninformed about the nature of the problem or the extent of the required correction. And in each case, the service provider has an incentive to overprovide to increase revenues, while the insured consumer has no incentive to countermand this overutilization tendency. Yet, no one seems to argue that car insurance should be subject to comprehensive federal regulation to assure consumer protection.

The authors note that the market for automobile insurance has developed mechanisms to respond to the problems created by the availability of insurance to the uninformed consumer. The same result could occur with health insurance. Crocker and Moran also acknowledge shortcomings in their analogy between health and automobile insurance. Coverage levels differ, with preventive care included in health insurance but not in car insurance. Unlike car insurance, with the upper limits of coverage set by the value of the car, there is no readily determinable upper boundary for the value of medical intervention in a human life.

Establishing that medical care is not unique, however, does not answer the questions that are raised by managed care. Crocker and Moran consider two related issues in a section of their chapter that discusses whether managed care is a panacea for medicine. They acknowledge that managed care enables the payer to obtain direct control over the providers and to create disincentives to overprovision of services that function also as incentives to underprovide. They pose the question of whether caregivers respond to managed-care incentives and, if so, whether patient care is compromised by those incentives. Second, they ask whether managed care can control costs over the long term. Their answers are, unavoidably, equivocal.

Like many of the authors, they decry the lack of available data. The scant evidence that is available suggests that providers do respond to managed-care incentives. But data on the larger question, whether the resultant reduction in services harms patients by withholding necessary care, are inconclusive. Early studies, conducted over short periods with a small number of plans when incentives were less extensive, suggest no difference in patient outcome. More recent studies, including those cited by Hurwit, suggest poorer outcomes in managed care than in fee-for-service medicine for patients with chronic conditions.

The authors also question whether managed care can achieve long-term cost control. Several studies suggest that, despite short-term gains, total health-care spending is similar under fee-for-service and managed-care systems. After considering a number of proposed legal and regulatory solutions and finding them wanting, the authors conclude that patients, providers, and payers will respond to economic incentives and that the solution lies in crafting economic incentives that respect behavioral realities.

Moving from market theory to market practice, the next two chapters are written on behalf of large purchasers of health-care benefits. In the first, Bruce E. Bradley and his coauthors at GM argue forcefully that market forces are preferable to regulation for the oversight of managed care. They assert that the demands of corporate purchasers in the marketplace will lead to a managed-care system that is fast, efficient, value driven, and evidence based. In sharp contrast to Anders and Noble and Brennan, whose legislative-based solutions rely on societal consensus through the democratic process, the authors of this chapter assert that the democratic process is flawed and the regulatory process unresponsive. The democratic process, they argue, suffers from the influence of political ideologies and of special interest groups. Regulation is slow to respond and, as a result, not based on current reliable evidence. Each author who supports market forces as the principal means of oversight for managed care echoes these dispersions of the legislative process and its output.

In comparison with regulation and the legislative process, the GM authors contend that market forces are faster and more efficient. Market forces provide an opportunity for evidence-based decisions that are flexible and adaptable as new data and performance measures are available. In addition, market forces are free of special interest groups and political influences. They assert that corporate purchasers will be driven by the diverse needs of their employee populations to design health benefit packages that meet those needs and to select high-quality managed-care plans. The authors maintain that corporate purchasers will respond to new information and hold managed-care organizations accountable through purchasing decisions and financial incentives. They also point out that GM has voluntarily adopted many aspects of the Consumer Bill of Rights that forms the basis for many proposed regulatory solutions. In essence, GM asserts that corporate purchasers will succeed where the democratic process has failed to protect the interests of their citizen-employees.

GM suggests that the government itself will be more effective as a purchaser than as a regulator. In his chapter, Bruce Bullen agrees and characterizes the state Medicaid program as a "prudent purchaser." Bullen seconds the arguments made by GM that purchasers can define and measure quality and can exert market leadership to achieve the optimal combination of cost and quality. In contrast to the authors who seek regulatory protection from state and federal governments, Bullen maintains that state Medicaid programs—themselves creatures of legislation—should not be impeded by misguided legislative consumer protections in their attempts to obtain value for the government's health-care dollar on behalf of Medicaid beneficiaries.

Not all purchasers are buying for large numbers of enrollees. How do small businesses use the marketplace to oversee managed-care plans for their employees? Margaret O'Kane, writing for the National Committee for Quality Assurance (NCQA), asserts that private accrediting agencies can leverage market pressure of small and large employers to promote quality in managed care.

O'Kane's chapter reflects partial consensus with both the advocates of regulation and those of market forces. She agrees with the proponents of regulation that health care is different. The key difference for her is that health-care services are not commodities of uniform price and quality. At the same time, she notes the limits of regulatory approaches. Like Bradley and his coauthors, she argues that regulation is slow and does not promote innovation and that regulatory processes are political and subject to influence by political pressures. She also observes that regulatory thresholds might set the bar too low and, therefore, might fail to offer significant protection to consumers or to encourage quality improvement by managed-care plans.

O'Kane contends that market forces will result in improved quality if two conditions are satisfied. First, economic incentives to improve quality must exist. Second, purchasers and consumers, when given adequate information about quality and performance, must select those organizations that provide high quality. NCQA, in its role as the lead accrediting agency for managed-care organizations, is working to develop quality measures and to make information available to purchasers and consumers. Nonetheless, the data do not establish conclusively that purchasers will respond to quality information by selecting high-quality plans. Presently, price is the principal competitive force in the managed-care marketplace. O'Kane believes that, when information is more extensive and more widely available, health plans will feel increased pressure to compete on quality and service. More data, and more reliable data, will be required to prove NCQA's hypothesis.

In chapter 11, the American Association of Health Plans (AAHP), the primary trade association for managed-care organizations, offers its own criticisms of regulatory initiatives. In a reprinted white paper, AAHP points out that managed-care organizations are already subject to extensive regulation from both the federal and state governments. If the definition of the term *regulation* is broadened to include any rules that govern behavior, managed-care organizations are also subject to oversight by purchasers and private accrediting agencies. The focus of AAHP's chapter is the predicted financial impact of four oft-cited regulatory proposals: increased exposure to malpractice liability; treatment of utilization review as the practice of medicine; prohibition of health plans from making medical necessity determinations; and any willing provider laws. The estimates are based on a study commissioned by AAHP and conducted by the Barents Group. Premium increases range from a low of 2.2 percent to a high of 8.6 percent for the various proposals. As a point of comparison, in 1998 the Congressional Budget Office estimated a 4 percent premium increase associated with the adoption of the Consumer Bill of Rights proposed by the President's Advisory Commission on Consumer Protection and Quality in the Health Care Industry. Karen Ignagni, president and chief executive officer of AAHP, disputed that figure in testimony before the Senate Health, Education, Labor, and Pensions Committee, arguing that it was too low.[18] The uncertainty of the costs of various consumer protection proposals only adds to the difficulty of addressing these issues.

In the final two chapters of the monograph, the reader returns to the subject of regulatory oversight of managed care. Frances Wallace, director of the Health Benefit Plans of the Michigan Insurance Bureau, describes her views on the role of a state department of insurance in the regulation of managed care. She proposes a federal-state collaboration for the oversight of managed care in which states bring to bear their historical expertise in insurance regulation and are permitted flexibility to experiment and respond to local needs, while the federal government lends its expertise to accomplish national objectives.

Professor Peter D. Jacobson's chapter concludes the monograph. He addresses a form of legal oversight that is frequently ignored in national health policy: the litigation of disputes between private parties. As the previous chapters illustrate, the dispute over the political or market forces tends to focus on legislation and regulation. The legal system, however, need not rely solely on statutes and regulations to achieve its ends. One alternative to regulation is the reliance on market forces to shape behavior and to permit individuals who may be harmed by the resultant activities to seek a remedy in court.[19] In addition, as private contract has become increasingly important in health-care coverage,[20] courts are called upon to interpret the terms of health insurance contracts and managed-care service agreements to resolve disputes between payer and patient or physician. Since lawyers advise their clients about proposed future activities based, in part, on resolved cases involving other parties, judicial opinions can influence future behavior of similarly situated parties under analogous facts and circumstances.

In his chapter, Jacobson explores the role of litigation between private parties in the regulation of managed-care organizations' activities, with a focus on their cost containment strategies. He identifies several important trends. First, his review of recent reported cases shows that courts are applying traditional liability doctrine to managed-care organizations. Second, he found no evidence that courts have systematically restricted cost containment innovations. Finally, he noted that courts have so far been unwilling to rely on public policy concerns as grounds to interfere with market-based managed-care initiatives. The net effect of the courts' reluctance to create new legal doctrine for managed care or to overturn private contract and market activities has been to leave accountability of managed-care organizations largely in the hands of legislatures. Jacobson's findings are consistent with the current focus on legislation that is reflected throughout the monograph.

A Cautionary Note

Too often those involved in the discussion about the proper means of oversight for managed care resort to simplistic or ideological solutions. The task of finding solutions to problems presented by the managed-care industry is made more difficult by contradictory perceptions about the existence, nature, and extent of those problems. An example found in this monograph is the disagreement about whether gag clauses were ever prevalent in contracts between managed-care organizations and physicians. State and federal legislation to prohibit something that did not exist remedies little, although it might score political points.

Even the "problem" to be solved is poorly defined. Is the issue the protection of patients, or must the needs of providers be addressed as well? Billi suggests that long-term adverse effects for health-care delivery could result from the exclusion of academic medical centers from managed-care plans, indicating that caregivers are ignored at society's peril. Even if the discourse should focus solely on the needs of patients, should it be limited to the protection of enrollees in managed care plans, or must it include the uninsured and the underinsured? Cleaveland's solution and Hurwit's proposal address the needs of the uninsured as well as the insured. GM's solution focuses on its employees. It would substitute the corporation motivated to make prudent purchasing decisions by its interest in attracting applicants and maintaining a healthy workforce for the democratic process with its political influences. Anders and Noble and Brennan, in contrast, would look to the democratic process as the means to develop responsive regulation. And what of employers without employee unions or market power? The small employer likely will not have the same clout with which to protect its employees as will GM or a state Medicaid program. NCQA asserts that it can leverage the influence of large and small employers to encourage managed-care plans to submit voluntarily to quality standards. Espousing an opposing view, Hurwit suggests that employer-as-purchaser is part of the problem of managed care, not part of the solution. Removing the consumer from the purchasing decision, in her view, makes managed care less responsive to patient needs. And reliance on market forces and volunteerism both ignores those without market power—the indigent and the chronically ill—and fails to provide a remedy for those harmed by managed-care practices.

Finally, the lack of available data exacerbates the onerous nature of the task. Contradictory perceptions could be resolved if data were available. Data might reveal that managed care is performing better, or worse, than the authors and the public assume. Without it, analysis resorts to theory and speculation.

Inevitably, our choice is not between an imperfect market system and a perfect legal system, nor is it a perfectly efficient market response against a costly, slow legislative answer. The solution to these difficult questions will be both more complex and less utopian. We will continue to struggle with the inevitable trade-off among quality, access, and cost and between and the needs and desires of individual patients and the requirements of patient populations. The true challenge is to determine what mix of market oversight and government intervention will yield quality cost-effective health care for the greatest number; restore consumer confidence in our health-care system; and encourage meaningful accountability by those who affect the health of the nation's citizens. The authors have shared their insights on achieving this goal and, in the course of doing so, have revealed much about the interests of major stakeholders in the health-care reform debate. We invite you to benefit from their views and to engage in this important dialogue.

NOTES

1. Theodore R. Marmor, "Forecasting American Health Care: How We Got Here and Where We Might Be Going," *J. Health Pol., Pol'y & L.* 23 (1998): 551, 561. Marmor notes that the term *managed care* conveys "competence and concern" but argues that in practice "managed care [has] mostly meant cutting back on payment levels, medical choices, and covered services."

2. William M. Sage, "Judicial Opinions Involving Health Insurance Coverage: Trompe L'Oeil or Window on the World," *Ind. L. Rev.* 31 (1998): 49, 51. Sage describes managed care as the convergence of coverage and care in a prepaid system.

3. Barbara A. Shickich, "Legal Consequences of the Health Maintenance Organization," in *Healthcare Facilities Law,* ed. Anne M. Dellinger (Boston, MA: Little, Brown & Co. 1991), 1051, 1052–60.

4. Thomas Mayer and Gloria Gilbert Mayer, "HMOs: Origins and Development," *N. Eng. J. Med.* 312 (1985): 590.

5. Vickie Y. Brown and Barbara R. Hartung, "Managed Care at the Crossroads: Can Managed Care Organizations Survive Government Regulation?" *Annals Health L.* 7 (1998): 25.

6. "Trends and Indicators in the Changing Health Care Marketplace," available through the Kaiser Family Foundation and at http://www.kff.ort/content/archive/1429.

7. For a discussion of antitrust laws and other factors that contributed to the shift in health care from a professional paradigm to a market paradigm, see James F. Blumstein, "Health Care Reform and Competing Visions of Medical Care: Antitrust and State Provider Cooperation Legislation," *Cornell L. Rev.* 79 (1994):1459.

8. 42 U.S.C. sections 300k–300n-6 (1974). The statute was repealed in 1986,

although some states have retained the basic health planning structure established under the act.

9. For example, N.C. Gen. Stat. section 131E–190 (1998) (penalty includes withholding of government funds for the new service, revocation, or suspension of license, civil monetary penalties, and ineligibility for state grants or other financial assistance).

10. Health Planning and Resources Development Amendments of 1979, Pub. Law. No. 96–79, 93 Stat. 592.

11. 42 U.S.C. section 300e–300e-17.

12. 29 U.S.C. section 1001–1461.

13. 42 U.S.C. section 300e–9. All employers subject to the Fair Labor Standards Act and employing twenty-five or more employees were required to offer their employees the option to enroll in a health maintenance organization, when a federal qualified health maintenance organization exercised its right to "mandate" that the employer do so. This section came to be known as the "dual-choice" provision.

14. The National Association of Insurance Commissioners first prepared model legislation in 1972.

15. U.S. Healthcare, Inc., purchased by Aetna Inc. in 1996 for $8.9 billion, is a case in point for the growth fostered by the federal HMO Act. Leonard Abramson started Pennsylvania-based U.S. Healthcare in the 1970s with family savings augmented by federal funding provided pursuant to the federal HMO Act. In the early 1980s, when Congress amended the act to encourage private investment in managed care, U.S. Healthcare became one of the first nonprofit corporations created under the incentives of the federal HMO Act to convert to equity ownership and for-profit status. In 1996, Abramson turned his formerly nonprofit HMO into a $920 million payoff. "Top Stories of '96: HMO Backlash, Quest for Quality," *Faulkner & Gray Medicine & Health*, Dec. 23, 1996.

16. Most commentators recognize that legal oversight is a matter of degree. The stock market, surely the epitome of the marketplace, is subject to extensive legal oversight. Few argue for a complete abdication by the legal system in health care. But see Richard Epstein, *Mortal Peril: Our Inalienable Right to Health Care?* (Reading, MA: Addison-Wesley Publishing Company, Inc., 1997).

17. Gail B. Agrawal, "Chicago Hope Meets the Chicago School," *Mich. L. Rev.* 96 (1998): 1793, 1818 n. 88 (a review of Mark A. Hall, *Making Medical Spending Decisions: The Law, Ethics, and Economics of Rationing Mechanisms*).

18. "Patients' Bill of Rights: Senate Fight Heats Up . . . Again," *The National Journal Group, Inc.*, Health Line (an on-line news service/publisher of health-related news), March 22, 1999.

19. This method would require an amendment to ERISA to be effective for a large segment of the population.

20. For an excellent discussion of the role of contract in health reform, see Clark Havighurst, *Health Care Choices: Private Contracts as Instruments of Health Reform* (Washington, D.C.: AEI Press, 1995).

CHAPTER 2

A National Overview

George Anders

For nearly two decades, the government's general role in the U.S. economy has been to pull back rather than to intercede. We have embraced deregulation as the best way to promote economic growth and innovation. Regulation of the private sector generally is seen as stifling and counterproductive, as much better at hobbling business than at safeguarding consumers.

In health care, however, things are different. Regulation has long been accepted as a cornerstone of medical and health insurance policy. The sweeping free-market advocacy of the Reagan-Bush years left much less of a mark on health care, where state and federal governments still finance at least one-third of all care. Hospitals, doctors, nurses, and ancillary services are subject to extensive government oversight. So, too, is the health insurance industry. In fact, since 1995, as managed care has become more prevalent, we have seen a rapidly intensifying interest in managed-care regulation among state legislators and insurance commissioners.

Why is regulation on the rise in health care, even as it wanes in other parts of the economy? I have asked that question frequently in my travels around the United States as an author and newspaper reporter. One of the most insightful answers came when I started researching the book that became *Health Against Wealth*.

I went to Harrisburg, Pennsylvania, in the spring of 1995 to meet Steve Male, the longtime head of health maintenance organization (HMO) regulation in that state. Male had a lot of time to spend with me. He had just been kicked out of his job by a governor who wanted someone friendlier to the insurance industry. So we sat in his backyard, as the spring afternoon turned

---

Editors' Note: Since the time that George Anders wrote this chapter, there has been continued activity in health-care regulation at both the state and national legislative levels. While the Omnibus Reconciliation Act referred to in this chapter was not enacted, similar legislation is being proposed at the time of this writing. In addition, several states have implemented new legislation, including some of the features mentioned by Anders. Although as of yet sweeping nationwide regulation of managed care, including fundamental changes in the ERISA preemption, has not occurred, it remains a hot legislative topic at both the national and state levels. To learn about the current status of legislation on a state-by-state and national level, see the web sites listed in appendix B.

into dusk, and we talked about what the role of regulation should be. Partway through our chat, he began to tell me how his views had changed over the years. In paraphrase, his fundamental message was this:

> When I started this job in the late 1970s, I felt my mission was to help HMOs grow. The whole medical establishment was so big, and arrogant, and expensive that we needed some sort of counterweight to them. Along came these little health plans that promised to watch over our premium dollars and make sure money was spent wisely. I did a lot back then to help them expand—and I was convinced I was doing the right thing. If the HMOs decided to negotiate lower hospital fees and not approve every surgery, well, we all knew that hospitals were charging frightening amounts and that some doctors were operating more often than they should.
>
> But now, I'm wondering if we went too far. I look at all the power that's been built up in the HMO industry. These aren't tiny health plans anymore. They are multibillion-dollar giants that can act with impunity.

In his view, HMOs had become marketing machines that did a great job of signing up members but that didn't always deliver the quality care that consumers had a right to expect. There seemed to be no limit to how much these health plans would lean on doctors and hospitals for cheaper rates and more restrictive contracts, in a business strategy that amounted to pursuing economic advantage without focusing on patients' needs. That changing balance of power, he believed, created an important role for someone, most likely the government, to police these health plans' behavior.

As I watch what is happening around the United States today, there is rapidly growing interest in supervising HMOs. In Washington, D.C., one sees only a handful of bills about certain flash point issues. But watch state legislatures—and important regulatory agencies such as the federal Health Care Financing Administration—and you will see a flurry of activity. Listen to consumer groups or medical societies and you will hear calls for even more regulation.

Fueling this regulatory push, I believe, is a variant of Steve Male's basic beliefs. When HMOs and other managed-care plans were a tiny movement on the edge of health care, everyone seemed inclined to let them write their own rules. Now managed care is about to become our national health policy, if it isn't so already. There were 58 million people enrolled in HMOs at the end of 1995;[1] that figure was expected to grow to 70 million members in 1996.[2] Another 91 million people were enrolled in looser forms of managed care, such as preferred provider organizations.[3] Put it all together and you can argue that managed care is displacing traditional indemnity health insurance in much the same way as the automobile displaced the horse-drawn carriage.[4] As managed care takes on such a prominent role, there is much greater concern about its impact on consumers and the medical system.

I would like to summarize for you the main regulatory initiatives that are under way. I will start by covering the battle that began in 1995 and then will look at what lies ahead. Most of these remarks will be from the perspective of my day job as a staff reporter at the *Wall Street Journal,* as I lay out facts without providing overly pointed interpretation. I will also briefly transform into my other incarnation as author and share with you some of the conclusions that I came to at the end of my book, especially as they relate to the role of regulation.

By one count, more than 400 managed-care related bills were introduced in state legislatures between 1995 and 1997. Leaving aside the bills that went nowhere, 40 states have enacted some new type of managed-care regulation.[5] Meanwhile, some federal courts have handed down rulings that could lead to a major rethinking of health plans' liability for medical consequences associated with insurance coverage decisions.[6]

In this fast-moving environment, we are lucky that two separate sets of experts, the Families USA Foundation and the HealthLine news service, have fastidiously tracked, sorted, and analyzed changes in managed-care regulation. Here is what they have observed:

- In 1995–96, twenty-eight states set standards for maternity lengths-of-stay, generally requiring insurers to offer forty-eight hours of coverage for uncomplicated vaginal births and ninety-six hours for cesarean sections, unless mother and doctor both opted for something shorter.[7] That stopped in its tracks efforts by managed-care plans and other insurers to trim coverage to as little as twenty-four hours. States involved include Illinois, New York, Ohio, and even South Dakota. Ultimately, the U.S. Congress itself passed legislation in this area;[8] it was signed into law by President Clinton in September 1996.
- Ten states passed legislation to address emergency care access.[9] The basic issue here involves some insurers' refusals to pay, after the fact, for emergency room (ER) visits that turned out to have been false alarms. Consumers and ER doctors argue that this is a harsh standard, because it is often difficult to know ahead of time whether frightening symptoms, such as severe chest pains, reflect a true emergency in the form of a heart attack or are simply caused by something less dramatic, namely indigestion. Make the payment standard too tough, these groups argue, and patients will be hesitant about coming to the ER with genuine emergencies, for fear that they will be stuck with the bill. The most common regulatory intervention here has been to require insurers to follow a more patient-friendly standard in deciding which emergency claims to pay. One such variant is known as the "prudent layperson" standard, which requires insurers to pay for emergency services if a prudent layperson would have reasonably believed that the symptoms involved could put his life or well-being in

immediate danger.[10] At least thirteen states have adopted this prudent layperson standard.[11]

- Eighteen states prohibited so-called gag clauses in doctors' contracts.[12] These clauses limit doctors' freedom to discuss certain managed-care issues with their patients. In the most extreme cases, such clauses bar doctors from telling sick patients about treatments that aren't covered by their health plans. More commonly, these clauses tell doctors that they aren't supposed to make disparaging comments about the managed-care plan to patients and that they aren't supposed to discuss with patients the contract details, such as financial incentives or penalties linked to how many patients get X rays, costly drugs, or emergency room visits. The HMO industry has defended some of these clauses as necessary for competitive reasons.[13] But physicians and consumer groups have argued that such provisions aren't in the public interest.[14]

- Twenty states have required managed-care plans to allow female members to have direct access to obstetricians and gynecologists (OB/GYNs). Previously, many plans used a "gatekeeper" system, in which primary care doctors had to write a referral to an OB/GYN before patients could get insurance coverage for such visits. That irritated many patients who felt that their need for such services was obvious and should not be hamstrung in managed-care bureaucracy. California and New York were the first states to act in this area, passing legislation in 1994;[15] other states, from Georgia to Oregon, have followed.[16]

- In addition, eighteen states passed laws or enacted regulations requiring HMOs to disclose more information to members. Among the areas for disclosure are policies on getting a specialist referral;[17] which prescription drugs are covered and not covered under a formulary;[18] how doctors are paid;[19] and what types of experimental therapy are covered and how those decisions are made.[20]

Probably the most comprehensive bills were passed in New York[21] and New Jersey;[22] their legislation included just about all of these elements.

Not every attempt to increase the regulation of managed care has succeeded. In chapter 12 of *Health Against Wealth,* I describe the 1995 defeat of a major bill in Texas dealing with managed-care issues.[23] The bill was strongly endorsed by the principal Texas physicians' organization but was actively opposed by employers, who argued that some of its provisions would push up their premiums. That argument ultimately carried the day with Gov. George W. Bush, who vetoed the bill. Although the bill was known as the Patient Protection Act, Governor Bush contended that it contained "too little protection for patients, and too much protection for special interests."

In California in 1996, two managed-care regulatory initiatives sponsored by nurses, health-care workers, and other people within the medical industry also failed. Those initiatives, known as Propositions 214 and 216, combined some proconsumer measures—such as greater health plan disclosure—with other provisions that were portrayed as job protection for various parts of the medical industry. Once again, insurers and employers banded together and successfully opposed the initiatives as being too costly.

Taken together, the Texas and California measures suggest that public appetite so far has been greatest for managed-care regulation on behalf of consumers. Public interest is significantly less for measures that seek to shore up the (now embattled) position of doctors, hospitals, and other medical providers.

So where do we go from here?

More proposals to regulate managed care are coming thick and fast. Some of them follow the pattern established in 1995–96, addressing fairly narrow coverage issues for specific medical needs. More commonly, though, proposed regulations are taking aim at the inner workings of managed-care plans—seeking to introduce new procedures for appeals, referrals, and other services so that consumers will be better served. Three areas taking shape as new regulatory battlegrounds include members' grievance and appeals rights, physicians' pay arrangements, and accountability of managed-care plans or employers for their mistakes.

Members' Grievance and Appeals Rights

Since the passage of the 1973 federal HMO Act, all federally chartered HMOs have been obligated to provide members with the right to file grievances and to appeal coverage decisions that they don't like. Leading consumer groups, however, have contended that grievance and appeals programs often aren't designed with the member in mind and can pose daunting obstacles to people seeking better care.

In 1997 the federal Health Care Financing Administration (HCFA), which oversees Medicare, first signaled its desire to improve appeals procedures for Medicare HMOs, which enroll more than 4.5 million people age sixty-five and older. Medicare HMOs have been allowed as much as sixty days to respond to members' appeals. Federal officials—and even many HMO executives—believe that timetable is too languid for many medical conditions. When a disease is worsening, decisions often can't be put on hold for two months, pending action on a coverage appeal. HCFA has published final regulations providing a much swifter, three-day standard for hearing appeals when the longer time would risk the beneficiary's life or health; more time is allowed only when complex issues require it.[24]

Because HCFA is the largest single purchaser of managed care, its decisions may prove to have a signaling effect on the rest of the marketplace, leading private employers to insist on managed-care appeals provisions that are "as good as Medicare."

Physicians' Pay Arrangements

In traditional health insurance, doctors collect extra revenue for each visit, test, or procedure. While that fee-for-service system encourages physicians to concentrate on their toughest cases, it has led to rapidly escalating costs and the risk of overtreatment—particularly as third-party employers or government programs have picked up most of the costs of care. Now, many managed-care plans are switching to various forms of capitation,[25] in which doctors are paid a fixed amount per patient per month regardless of how sick or healthy each patient might be. Those arrangements encourage physicians to make decisions within a budget. Capitation can encourage more attention to preventive care and management of chronic diseases, as doctors spend a little up front to avoid bigger costs later on. But capitation also raises new risks of undertreatment and physician redlining, or refusal to accept sick patients whose care needs might be a drain on a doctor's budget.[26]

Capitation oversight is a new field, and regulators in many cases are still learning what questions to ask. As capitation gains ground, though, consumer groups, doctors, and regulators are likely to be more active. HCFA already has imposed regulations on physician incentive plans in which doctors' groups accept significant financial risks, so that physicians don't inadvertently trap themselves in a situation where they risk insolvency if they cater to a few sick patients' medical needs.[27] Consumer groups, meanwhile, have been pushing for greater disclosure of physicians' pay arrangements under capitation, particularly if health plans offer bonuses linked to frugal use of certain services. Health plans have so far resisted such disclosure.

Accountability of Managed-Care Plans or Employers for Their Mistakes

Currently, many big companies don't actually buy health insurance for their workers; they assume the insurance risk themselves and merely hire a managed-care company to administer the program. When that happens, it is difficult to pin down anyone directly responsible for a coverage denial that may have led to a bad medical outcome. Patients who have tried suing managed-care plans for negligence in state court have found their lawsuits moved to federal court, with most of their claims then dismissed under what is known as the ERISA preemption. ERISA is the landmark 1974 pension law that has been interpreted to mean that you can't sue an employer-run health plan for damages.

Texas enacted a bill to permit lawsuits alleging health-plan negligence.[28] That would mean HMOs could be sued for sizable damages by members who attribute medical disasters to the health plan's restrictive rules. Patients and doctor groups say this is a needed reform that would create a powerful deterrent against undercare. Other states are considering similar legislation.[29] Health plans and big corporations don't want to see the ERISA preemption disappear; they say it would jack up their costs and expose them to all sorts of unwarranted suits every time they tried to make a medical decision.

So far, no one has overturned the ERISA preemption, but some recent federal court rulings have suggested that ERISA's relevance to health care ought to be reexamined. Many of these reforms were packaged together in an omnibus federal bill that was introduced by Sen. Edward Kennedy (D—Mass.) and Rep. John Dingell (D—Mich.). Their bill, known as the Health Insurance Bill of Rights Act, would ban gag rules, require easier access to emergency care, require primary access to obstetricians and gynecologists for women needing those services, and improve health-plan members' access to clinical trials. Their bill also would nudge HMOs to adhere to uniformly high standards on some governance issues, notably better dispute resolution. It also would require clearer disclosure ahead of time about the procedures involved if members want a referral to a specialist, a renowned hospital, or a special diagnostic test.

Over the next few years, the progress of this new regulatory drive will be governed by the ability—or inability—of consumers, doctors, employers, and insurers to reach consensus on what must be done. Often, discussion of managed-care regulation turns into a tug-of-war. Consumer groups and physicians advocate more regulation; employers and insurers oppose such moves as too costly. In such settings, change is intermittent and convulsive.

There are encouraging signs, however, that all four of the main interest groups may be able to work together. In Ohio, a bill on managed-care regulation was jointly endorsed by the state medical association and by Kaiser Permanente, the giant HMO, which is active in that state. In Washington, the main managed-care trade group, the American Association of Health Plans (see chapter 11), has lent cautious support to some proposals for improved HMO governance. And in California, major employer purchasing coalitions are looking for ways to work more effectively with doctors and consumer groups.

Such meetings of the minds are encouraging news. Health care is one of the few industries where hands-on, day-to-day regulation is inevitable and perhaps even valuable. While market forces can help us get a faster computer chip, a funnier movie, or a tastier chocolate-chip cookie, the consequences of unregulated health care or medical insurance are much less palatable. In health insurance, consumers and employers must make purchasing decisions months—or even years—before they know their actual medical needs. Treatment decisions often arise at times of great anxiety and vulnerability. And not all customers are alike. Without some mechanism to broaden coverage, insurers will be tempted to sign up the healthy, shun the sick, and avoid paying out any more of the premium dollar for claims than they absolutely have to.

It is little wonder that when consumers are asked which industries they trust the most, and which ones they regard as delivering the best value for their money, health care and medical insurance rank near the bottom of the list. Anyone approaching the subject of HMO regulation must hope that it is possible to improve things. Managed care, in theory, has a great deal to offer the American public. It can help lower costs, make sure resources are allocated more intelligently, and lead to coordinated, well-planned care that would be a major improvement from what can often be a haphazard system of treatment. But the managed-care industry today is a long way from living up to that potential. Without some sort of mechanism to point plans in the right direction, there is a risk that competition in the managed-care industry will degrade to some version of Gresham's law, where the bad plans drive out the good.

For that reason alone, the subject of managed-care regulation is timely, compelling, and full of promise.

NOTES

This paper was presented in the summer of 1997 and subsequently edited and annotated in May 1999.

1. See American Association of Health Plans, *1995–1996 AAHP HMO and PPO Trends Report* (visited Jan. 31, 1998, at http://www.aahp.org/services/research /0613rep.htm).

2. Ibid.

3. Ibid.

4. See generally John K. Iglehart, "The American Health Care System: Managed Care," *New Eng. J. Med.* 327 (1992): 742–43 ("The reality is that this new model has rapidly emerged as a dominant one in the American health care system.").

5. Families USA reports that forty states had passed laws affecting HMOs by the end of 1996 that were intended to protect consumers. See Families USA, *HMO Consumers at Risk: States to the Rescue* (visited Jan. 6, 1998, at http://www.familiesusa .org/hmocon2.html).

6. See, e.g., *Herdrick v. Pegram*, 154 F.3d 362 (7th Cir. 1998) reversed, 120 S.Ct. 2143 (2000); *Dukes v. U.S. HealthCare, Inc.*, 57 F.3d 350 (3d Cir. 1995).

7. See Families USA, *HMO Consumers at Risk: States to the Rescue* (visited Jan. 6, 1998, at http://www.familiesusa.org/hmocon2.html). Statute provisions vary, but most set minimum coverage levels and allow exceptions when the doctor and patient agree that a shorter stay would be appropriate. Some also mandate follow-up care when mothers and newborns are sent home early. See, e.g., Ala. Code § 27–48–2 (1996), Conn. Gen. Stat. Ann. § 38a–503(c) (West 1997), Fla. Stat. Ann. § 641.31(18)(b)(West 1997), Ga. Code Ann. § 33–24–58.1 (1996), 215 Ill. Comp. Stat. Ann. 5/356S (West 1997), Ind. Code Ann. § 27–8–25–5 (Burns 1996), Iowa Code Ann. § 514C.12 (West

1996), Kan. Stat. Ann. § 40–2, 160 (1996), Ky. Rev. Stat. Ann. § 304.17A–145 (Banks-Baldwin 1997), Me. Rev. Stat. Ann. Tit. 24A § 4234-B (West 1997) (health maintenance organizations), Md. Code Ann. Health-Gen. § 19–1305.4 (Supp. 1995), Mass. Regs. Code tit. 211 § 48.01 et seq. (1996), Minn. Stat. Ann. § 62A–0411 (West 1997).

8. See the Newborns' and Mothers' Health Protection Act of 1996, 29 U.S.C. § 1185 (1996). This act is intended to fill gaps in the state laws and to apply to out-of-state health plans and those for which state law is preempted by ERISA. Like many state statutes, the act mandates coverage for forty-eight hours following a vaginal birth and ninety-six hours after a cesarean section, unless the attending physician and mother determine that a shorter period of stay is appropriate.

9. See Families USA, *HMO Consumers at Risk: States to the Rescue* (visited Jan. 6, 1998, at http://www.familiesusa.org/hmocon2.html_).

10. The Board of the American College of Emergency Physicians adopted its own "prudent layperson" definition of emergency services in 1994. See Families USA, *HMO Consumers at Risk: States to the Rescue* (visited Jan. 6, 1998, at http://www.familiesusa .org/hmocon2.html_). See, e.g., Ga. Code Ann. §§ 31–11–80, 31–11–81, 31–11–82 (1996). This law defines "emergency condition" as:

> any medical condition of a recent onset and severity . . . that would lead a prudent layperson, possessing an average knowledge of medicine and health, to believe that his or her condition, sickness, or injury is of such a nature that failure to obtain immediate medical care could result in:
>
> (A) placing the patient's life in serious jeopardy;
> (B) serious impairment to bodily functions; or
> (C) serious dysfunction of any bodily organ or part.

11. See, e.g., Alaska Stat. § 08.64.380 (Michie 1997), Ark. Code Ann. § 20–9–309 (Michie 1995), Cal. Health & Safety Code § 1317 (West 1997), Idaho Code § 41–3903 (1997), Md. Code Ann., Health-Gen. I § 19–701 (1995), Minn. Stat. § 62Q–55 (1997), Mo. Ann. Stat. § 354.400 (West 1997), 1997 Nev. Stat. 695G.170, N.Y. Ins. Law § 3216(I)(9) (McKinney 1997), N.C. Gen. Stat. § 58–3–190 (1997), Tex. Ins. Code Ann. § 20A.02 (West 1997), Va. Code Ann. § 38.2–4300 (Michie 1997).

12. See e.g., Colo. Rev. Stat. Ann. § 10–16–121(1) (West 1997) (requiring contract provision that neither the provider nor the insurance carrier may be prohibited from expressing disagreement with decisions of the other). See also Ariz. Rev. Stat. Ann. § 20–1061 (West 1997), Cal. Bus. & Prof. Code § 2056.1 (West 1997), Del. Code Ann. Tit. 18 § 6407 (1996), Ga. Code Ann. § 33–20A–7 (1997), Me. Rev. Stat. Ann. Tit. 24–A § 4303 (West 1996), Md. Code Ann. Ins. § 15–116 (1997), Mass. Gen. Laws. Ann. Ch. 176G, § 6 (West 1997), N.H. Rev. Stat. Ann. § 420-B:12(IX) (1996), N.Y. Ins. Law § 4803(e) (McKinney 1997), 40 Pa. Cons. Stat. Ann. § 1584 (West 1997), R.I. Gen. Laws § 27–41–14.1 (1997), Tex. Ins. Code Ann. § 20A18A (West 1997), Wash. Rev. Code Ann. § 40.43.075 (West 1997).

13. See Karen Ignagni, "What Managed Care Plans Can Do to Counter the Horror Stories," 6 *Managed Care Week,* June 17, 1996, available at 1996 WL 8690222 at *2–3. Ignagni explains that "anti-disparagement" clauses are intended to have providers settle disputes with the health plan through contractual grievance provisions rather than reacting by criticizing the plan to patients. The purpose of "confidentiality clauses" is to keep providers from disclosing compensation arrangements.

14. For the position of physicians and other providers on gag clauses, see e.g., American Academy of Family Physicians, "Gag Clauses in Managed Care Contracts" (visited Apr. 5, 1998, at http://www.aafp.org/managed/gagrule.html). For the position of consumer groups, see e.g., Families USA, "Medicaid Managed Care Protections Needed" (visited Apr. 5, 1998, at http://www.familiesusa.org/mem05282.html).

15. See, e.g., Cal. Health & Safety Code § 1367.69 (West 1997).

16. See, e.g., Ala. Code § 27–49–4 (1996), Ark. Code Ann. § 23–99–406 (Michie 1997), Del. Code Ann. Tit. 18 § 3342 (1997) (individual policies), Del. Code Ann. Tit. 18 § 3356 (1997) (group policies), Fla. Stat. Ann. § 641.19 (West 1997), Ga. Code Ann. § 33–24–59 (1997), Idaho Code § 41.3915 (1997) La. Rev. Stat. Ann. § 22:215.17 (West 1997), Md. Code Ann., Health-Gen. I § 19–706 1997), Miss. Code Ann. § 83–41–217 (1997), Mo. Ann. State. § 354.618 (West 1997), Neb. Rev. Stat. § 44–786 (1997), Tex. Ins. Code Ann. § 21.53D (West 1997), Va. Code Ann. § 38.2–3407.11 (Michie 1997), W. Va. Code § 33–25A–2 (1997).

17. See, e.g., N.Y. Public Health Law § 4408 (McKinney 1997).

18. See, e.g., Ark. Code Ann. § 23–99–413 (Michie 1997), Colo. Rev. Stat. Ann. § 26–4–117 (West 1997), Ga. Code Ann. § 33–21–13 (1997). Some states are also requiring written procedures for patients to obtain nonformulary drugs without penalty or delay. See, e.g., Ark. Code Ann. § 23–409 (Michie 1997), Colo. Rev. Stat. Ann, § 26 4 115 (1997), Ga. Code Ann. § 33–21–13 (1997)

19. See, e.g., N.Y. Public Health Law § 4408 (McKinney 1997) (requiring disclosure of a description of methodologies used by the HMO to reimburse providers).

20. See, e.g., *Hendricks v. Central Reserve Life Insurance Co.* (39 F.3d 507 (4th Cir. 1994)), which allowed the plan's denial of coverage for HDC/PSCR for small cell lung cancer because the treatment was considered experimental; and *Fuja v. Benefit Trust Life Insurance* (18 F.3d 1405 (7th Cir. 1994)), which denied coverage for HDC/ABMT for breast cancer because the treatment was deemed experimental. See generally Mark A. Hall and Gerard F. Anders, "Health Insurers' Assessment of Medical Necessity," *U. Pa. L. Rev.* 140 (1992): 1637, 1654–57 (giving parameters of "experimental" and difficulties of enforcing contract terms when issues of health versus money arise).

21. See N.Y. Public Health Law § 4408 (McKinney 1997). The Managed Care Consumers' Bill of Rights took effect on April 1, 1997. New requirements cover the adequacy of primary care and specialist networks, the prohibition of physician gag clauses, the standardization of "medically necessary" treatment determinations, and the establishment of appeals procedures for plan decisions.

22. The Health Care Quality Act mandates a point-of-service option for all managed-care plans that would cover out-of-network care. MCOs are required to describe covered services to members with clarity; gag clauses are prohibited from provider contracts; and patients are given the right to appeal denials of coverage to an independent board of experts. Plans are required to disclose financial incentives to providers and established plan standards for customary waiting times and appointments. Doctors are also granted the right to appeal early termination of their contracts to a three-physician panel.

23. House Bill 2766. The bill, introduced by Republican representative John Smithee and Democratic senator Jim Turner, was drafted by Texas doctors who wanted to "fix" a variety of shortcomings in managed care. It called for better guarantees of due process before doctors could be fired from HMO networks, better access for patients to medical "centers of excellence," approval of coverage for emergency-room visits within

sixty minutes of contact with the company, more extensive HMO disclosure about the payments made to doctors and the quality of care they provided, and a requirement that large employers offer more than just an HMO to workers. See George Anders, *Health Against Wealth* (Boston, MA: Houghton Mifflin Co.) 217–18.

24. The rule was published on April 30, 1997. See 62 Fed. Reg. 23368 (1997). Consumer advocates claim that the final rule is flawed because, among other reasons, it leaves to the HMO the decision of whether the appeal is to be expedited or conducted under the standard process.

25. "As of February 1995, of 340 HMOs reporting 70% paid at least some primary care physicians through capitation: 50% did the same for specialist physicians." Emily Friedman, "Capitation, Integration, and Managed Care: Lessons from Early Experiments," *JAMA* 275 (1996): 957.

26. See Steven S. Sharfstein, "Prospective Cost Allocations for the Chronic Schizophrenic Patient," *Schizophrenia Bull* 17 (1992): 395; Jinnet B. Fowles et al., "Taking Health Status into Account When Setting Capitation Rates: A Comparison of Risk-Adjustment Methods," *JAMA* 276 (1996): 1316–1317.

27. 42 C.F.R. § 417.479 (1998).

28. Tex. Civ. Prac. & Rem. Code §§ 88.001–.003 (1998). The bill was challenged on ERISA preemption grounds and held preempted in part *(Corporate Health Ins. v. Texas Dept. of Ins.,* 12 F.Supp. 2d 597 (S.D. Tx. 1998)). (Affd in part, den'd in part, 215 F.3d 526 (5th. Cir. 2000); petn. for cert. filed (October 24, 2000)).

29. The Florida legislature passed a managed-care liability bill (HB 1853), but it was vetoed by Gov. Lawton Chiles. See Bureau of National Affairs' *Health Law Reporter* 851, June 6, 1996. Georgia and California have also passed managed-care liability laws.

CHAPTER 3

The Stages of Managed-Care Regulation: Developing Better Rules

Alice A. Noble and Troyen A. Brennan

Recent developments in the regulation of managed care reflect an industry that is very much at a crossroads. Nearly 75 percent of U.S. workers with health insurance now receive that coverage through some form of managed-care organization, as compared to 30 percent a decade ago (Jensen et al. 1997). Some predict that within the next ten years all insured Americans will be enrolled in managed-care plans (Bureau of National Affairs 1995). Consistent with this prediction, the federal government is moving toward making managed care an ever more significant form of health-care delivery for Medicare and Medicaid recipients (Kinney 1996; Iglehart 1997; Lamphere et al. 1997).

However, now that costs appear to be under control and more people are enrolled, the quality of the health care provided by managed-care organiza-

Editors' note: A version of this article was published in 1999 in volume 24 of the Journal of Health Politics, Policy and Law. Since that time, the stages of managed-care regulation have continued to evolve, and the observations made by Professors Noble and Brennan have proved prophetic.

Recent Supreme Court cases may have opened the door for greater state oversight through traditional state-law theories. State attorneys-general have begun to take a more active role in the oversight of managed-care organizations, as exemplified by a recent highly publicized settlement agreement reached between the state of Texas and Aetna Inc. And, the private plaintiffs' bar, in the wake of its recent victories against the tobacco industry, has instituted a series of class-action suits against managed-care organizations. Meanwhile, federal and state courts continue to struggle with the proper scope of preemption of state laws by federal law. These developments suggest that in the current stage of managed-care regulation private and public litigation may play a substantial role.

At the same time, managed care has continued to be a rich subject for state legislative and regulatory intervention. Several states, notably Georgia and California, have followed the lead of Texas in enacting legislation to expand the liability of managed-care organizations. Federal legislation, also, continues to loom large with competing bills aimed at protecting the rights of enrollees in managed-care organizations introduced in the early days of President George W. Bush's administration.

Managed care as an industry also continues to evolve in response to market pressures, making its regulation something of a moving target for both the legislative and judicial branches of federal and state government. Many of the problems identified by Professors Noble and Brennan in this chapter continue, and many of their recommendations are yet to be achieved.

tions is being questioned (Gosfield 1997). According to a recent survey by the Kaiser Family Foundation and Harvard University, 51 percent of individuals surveyed believe managed care has lowered the quality of care for the sick (Blendon et al. 1998).

The belief that market forces alone can create an environment that fosters quality health care at reduced cost is eroding. As a result, since early in this decade states have passed legislation at unprecedented rates aimed at ameliorating physician and consumer dissatisfaction (Miller 1997; see also chapter 2). Many HMO statutes passed in the 1970s are being reexamined in view of the explosive growth of managed care, organizational changes, and, perhaps most significant, the perceived dissatisfaction among consumers. The federal government has also become active in this area, most notably the Health Care Financing Administration. In addition, Congress has considered a number of managed-care bills. Thus a "consumer backlash" is shaping the managed-care debate at both the state and federal levels (Bodenheimer 1996; Budetti 1997).

While these state-based initiatives were originally adopted in an "à la carte" fashion with significant variation from state to state, a pattern began to emerge, as legislation came to reflect more settled expectations of what managed care should provide. This pattern of legislation will likely continue to be on the "menu" of proconsumer legislation in many states. Various proposals before Congress contain many consumer protections from this menu as well.

Other recent developments, although not as widely publicized, are also subtly molding this evolution of managed care. Examples of such influences include calls for greater oversight of risk-bearing entities and of physician incentive plans, as well as congressional proposals for a broader-based and more uniform regulatory scheme for managed care. Also, federal preemption of state oversight, particularly by the Employee Retirement Income Security Act (29 U.S.C. sections 1001–1461), has created uncertainty as to the role of state versus federal regulation. Finally, statutes attempting to impose liability on managed-care plans for negligent utilization review and patient care cannot be ignored. We submit that, as the immediate backlash against managed care gives way, these developments, taken together, may signal a new stage in which proposals with the potential to make a more subtle and long-lasting impact are emerging.

A growing awareness that quality problems are not unique to managed care may also serve to moderate reflexive, anti-managed-care regulation. Two influential groups, the Institute of Medicine National Roundtable on Health Care Quality (Chassin et al. 1998) and the President's Advisory Commission on Consumer Protection and Quality in the Health Care Industry (Advisory Commission 1998), have concluded that quality problems of overuse, underuse, and misuse of health care occur with the same frequency in both fee-for-service and managed-care systems. Thus managed-care quality can be seen as part of a more generalized focus on quality problems that has emerged as concerns about rising health-care costs have abated (Chassin et al. 1998).

From the vantage point of this managed-care crossroads, we describe and analyze the stages of managed-care regulation. We identify four stages. This analysis will focus upon how well each stage meets what we deem the most salient objectives of a reasonably functioning health-care system: quality care, access, and cost containment. We will also evaluate the responsiveness of proposed regulation. Because market forces continue to be important to the balance of cost containment and quality, regulation that can adapt to fit the new forms and influences in health-care delivery without stifling innovation, that is, "responsive regulation," is essential (Brennan and Berwick 1996).

After some background discussion, the following sections consider stages of managed-care regulation, from the relative calm of the 1970s to the more tempestuous atmosphere of the present. We will then discuss these developments, the trends in regulation that they may portend, and offer our recommendations for improving regulatory oversight.

Background: The Context of Managed-Care Regulation

The hallmark of managed care is the integration of health-care finance and delivery. By combining these functions, the managed-care organization can monitor quality across a population and provide incentives, both rule based and financial, to maintain the health of enrollees while controlling costs. Managed care first gained prominence in the 1970s. At that time rising health-care costs, emerging theories supporting deregulation, and a greater deference to market forces in health insurance and health-care delivery enhanced the appeal of managed care that, by definition, would address the risk of excess medical expenditures (Enthoven 1993). Also, the science of quality and outcomes measures and information technology had matured to such a point that the ability of managed care to provide internal incentives that would promote quality health care and discourage costly inappropriate care now seemed feasible.

Given the desire to promote HMO development and the incentives inherent in the HMO structure to self-regulate, governmental regulation of managed care was initially limited and deferential to the market. Throughout the 1990s, however, we saw an increase in governmental activism in managed-care regulation. Today it is recognized that market forces, the government, and private sector initiatives (such as accrediting bodies) all have a role in managed-care regulation (Enthoven and Singer 1997; Moran 1997).

This governmental activism emanates from both the state and federal levels, creating some tensions and uncertainties for regulators and for the regulated entities. Because this federal-state dynamic can be influential in the development and implementation of regulation, the following discussion of the federal and state division of labor may provide some insight into the regulatory developments we discuss in the following sections.

Under the U.S. Constitution, the scope of federal power is defined by certain enumerated powers. The Tenth Amendment provides that whatever powers are not delegated to the federal government are reserved to the states, or to the people. According to the operation of the Supremacy Clause, Art. VI, when Congress acts pursuant to one of its enumerated powers, such law is the "supreme Law of the Land," capable of preempting state law. Traditionally, health-care regulation was regarded as the province of the states. However, over the past thirty years the federal government has increasingly regulated the field (see Parmet 1993). This is significant because where Congress has expressed an intent to occupy a field exclusively, state laws, whether consistent or inconsistent with federal law, are preempted. Moreover, if Congress has not actively legislated in the preempted area, states are preempted from filling that regulatory vacuum. The operation of ERISA, a federal statute adopted pursuant to the congressional commerce clause power that expressly preempts state law, has created just such a vacuum (Chirba-Martin and Brennan 1994).

ERISA was enacted in 1974 to provide for national uniform administration of employee pension and health plans through federal legislation and to promote the growth of these private plans by freeing them from state laws, which unnecessarily complicate employee benefit administration. In order to achieve the goals of uniformity and plan autonomy, ERISA specifically preempts state laws that "relate to" any employee benefit plan (29 U.S.C. sec. 1144(b)(2)(B)).

A limitation on federal preemption can be found in ERISA. Consistent with the McCarran-Ferguson Act (Pub. Law 79–15, codified at 15 U.S.C.S. 1011–15 (Lexis 1998)), which was enacted in 1945 to preserve the state power to regulate the business of insurance, state laws that regulate insurance are exempted from preemption by ERISA's "savings clause" (29 U.S.C. sec. 1144(b)(2)(B)). However, the "business of insurance" left to the states by the McCarran-Ferguson Act and the ERISA savings clause has been interpreted very narrowly by the Supreme Court (see *Group Life & Health Insurance Co. v. Royal Drug,* 440 U.S. 205 (1979)). These developments have been reviewed in great detail elsewhere (Mariner 1996; Farrell 1997).

This insurance exception is limited, however, by the "deemer clause." Under the deemer clause, an ERISA self-insured plan cannot be deemed to be in the business of insurance for the purposes of state regulation. At the time of the enactment of ERISA only a small number of large employers had begun to self-insure. However, the deemer clause has provided a strong incentive for employers to avoid more burdensome state regulations by self-insuring. Today it is estimated that of the approximately 150 million Americans enrolled in ERISA plans approximately 55 million are enrolled in self-insured plans.

The ERISA vacuum has created a patchwork system that prevents state law regulating managed care from being uniformly enforced and deprives ERISA health plan enrollees of the benefit of state-enacted consumer protections and other legal remedies (Farrell 1997; Mariner 1996; Polzer and Butler 1997). For example, many managed-care regulations, such as disclosure requirements, utilization review standards, solvency requirements, mandated benefit laws, and grievance procedure requirements, are arguably preempted as "relating to" ERISA plans. Also, some courts interpret ERISA as preventing patients from bringing malpractice actions against managed care or utilization review organizations.

In a departure from this laissez-faire approach of ERISA, as well as from the federal deference to state insurance regulation, Congress has taken a more active role in some aspects of health insurance regulation. The most significant of these are the Consolidated Omnibus Budget Reconciliation Act of 1985 (COBRA), which provides for the continuation of employee health coverage benefits in certain circumstances, and the Health Insurance Portability and Accountability Act of 1996 (HIPAA), which requires insurance portability from job to job (see Furrow et al. 1997). Unlike ERISA, the COBRA and HIPAA regulatory schemes acknowledge state expertise by setting minimum federal standards to be enforced by the states.

These examples of federalism demonstrate the uncertainty of the federal-state division of labor. Moreover, the question of federal and state roles, as demonstrated by ERISA, may involve a question not only of jurisdiction but of significant policy differences as well. With this background in mind, we consider the stages of managed-care regulation.

Stages of Managed-Care Regulation

The First Stage: Regulation in the 1970s and 1980s

As discussed elsewhere in some detail, the regulation of managed care is now more than twenty-five years old (Brennan and Berwick 1996). The promotion of managed care began in earnest with the federal HMO Act of 1973 (42 U.S.C. section 300e et seq.). Much of the growth of managed care can be traced to the incentives contained within this federal HMO Act (see chapter 1).

The HMO Act did not completely preempt state regulation. Thus states were equally active in managed-care regulation, creating a variety of laws to oversee the financial health of the managed-care industry. Following a number of relatively high-profile insolvencies in the managed-care industry in the mid-1980s, rules regarding reserving and reporting of financial statistics that had previously only applied to traditional insurers were extended to the managed-care industry (Brennan and Berwick 1996).

There were also efforts to increase information for potential beneficiaries at the time that they enrolled in HMOs. States extended physician credentialing responsibilities to managed-care organizations (Kopit and Lutes 1993). Related to this, managed-care organizations were required to demonstrate that they had sufficient numbers of participating physicians in each specialty and that they were geographically dispersed in reasonable proximity of enrollees (Moran 1997). Health carriers also had to certify that they had means for continuing to check the efficiency of their networks. Health plans were also expected to have specific grievance procedures in place, including expedited review for specific rapidly developing illnesses (Physician Payment Review Commission 1995).[1]

Drawing on traditional modes of regulation, such as reporting, disclosure, credentialing, and due process requirements, in addition to borrowing regulatory techniques from other industries, states addressed quality and access concerns by devising new rules for the new industry. This first stage of regulation has demonstrated staying power. Indeed many of the requirements have been incorporated into private regulatory programs, such as the National Committee for Quality Assurance oversight mechanisms.[2] Also, the National Association of Insurance Commissioners (NAIC) (1996) has consolidated many of the elements of these regulations into model acts that have been closely examined by many states (NAIC 1996a).

As states continued to rely upon, to modify, and to develop these early regulatory structures, other influences emerged, most notably a perceived consumer dissatisfaction. Fueled in part by growing provider (primarily hospital and doctor) concern about the effect of managed care on income, pressure increased on state legislatures to address the "evils" of managed care.

The Second Stage: Anti-Managed-Care Regulations of the Mid-1990s

The second stage of regulation of managed care was marked by a surge in the number of managed-care laws, as state legislators responded swiftly to the growing consumer backlash against managed care. These measures were typically narrowly targeted and reflexive, with no discernible regulatory game plan or uniformity, yet reflecting an anti-managed-care proclivity (Bodenheimer 1996; Bureau of National Affairs 1995, 1996a). Examples of such laws include maternity length-of-stay bills, bans of gag clauses, and mandated access to specialists. Criticism has been leveled at the incremental or à la carte approach to regulation as being dominated by anecdotes of "horrors" committed by HMOs and leaving gaps in the regulation of health plan quality (Horvath and Snow 1996; Riley 1997).

The most prominent reform mechanism that captured the anti-managed-care sentiment of this stage of managed-care regulation was the any willing provider (AWP) law. Such laws, enacted in approximately twenty-three states, required managed-care plans to accept any provider willing to accept the terms and conditions of participation in the plan (Laudicina et al. 1998). The most common AWP statutes are aimed at opening panels to pharmacists, but some

AWP laws apply to most or all providers (Laudicina et al. 1998, appendix). Because AWP laws seek to fundamentally alter managed-care techniques, such as the gatekeeping function and limited provider panels, they prompted an unlikely alliance between business and the managed-care industry in lobbying against them with apparent success (Bureau of National Affairs 1996c). While thirteen such laws were passed in 1993 and 1994, as of 1998 roughly a handful of additional AWP laws had been enacted. (Bureau of National Affairs 1996c; Jaklevic 1996; Laudicina et al. 1998). Although fifteen states considered AWP laws in 1999 (Bureau of National Affairs 1998), ERISA case law has demonstrated that preemption poses a serious hurdle to the viability of such measures.

Decisions by the United States Court of Appeals for the Fifth Circuit, holding that AWP laws of Louisiana and Texas were preempted by ERISA, may at least partially explain the decline in state passage of AWP laws. These cases—*Cigna Healthplan v. State of Louisiana*, 82 F. 2d 642 (5th Cir.), cert. denied, 117 S. Ct. 387 (1996), and *Texas Pharmacy Association v. Prudential Insurance Company*, 105 F. 3d 1035 (5th Cir.), cert. denied, 118 Sup. Ct. 75 (1997)—both held that the AWP laws in question "relate to" ERISA plans because the statute eliminates the choice of one method of structuring benefits by prohibiting plans from contracting with networks that exclude any willing provider.[3]

States have given these holdings much weight, especially since they were decided shortly after the United States Supreme Court opinion in *New York Conference of Blue Cross and Blue Shield Plans v. Travelers*, 514 U.S. 645 (1995), which was expected to make such findings of ERISA preemption less likely. In *Travelers* the Supreme Court considered the preemptive reach of the "relate to" clause. The Court rejected a literal interpretation of this clause as being essentially limitless in breadth (see Jordan 1996). Speaking generally, after *Travelers* the door is slightly ajar for state regulation. What will fit through this opening is not certain and is subject to interpretation by the courts.

The subsequent Supreme Court case of *DeBuono v. NYSA-ILA and Clinical Services Fund*, 117 S. Ct. 1747 (1997), affirmed and elaborated the *Travelers* holding.[4] Relying on both *Travelers* and *DeBuono*, the United States Court of Appeals for the Eighth Circuit in *Prudential Insurance Company v. National Park Medical Center*, 154 F. 3d 812 (8th Cir. 1998), held that ERISA preempted the AWP law in question.

AWP laws purport to put a premium on the regulatory objective of access. Some would argue that such laws would increase access while jeopardizing quality and cost, since limited provider panels may allow plans greater control over the quality of physicians and their productivity. However, the market may have a greater influence here than state regulations. A 1995 study found that an equal number of health plans were opening their panels to all providers meeting credentialing requirements as were limiting their panels (Gold et al. 1995). As Berenson notes, consumer demand for choice of physician continues to be a powerful force in the market (1997).

The Third Stage: A Legislative Pattern Emerges

In stage three, specific trends have taken shape. States have begun to emulate one another with regard to certain generic types of oversight of managed care. In doing so, states seem to be choosing more narrow battles, such as gag clauses and patient access, and regulating rather than mandating provider selection.

The following sections describe what appear to be the most salient trends of state regulation. As will be seen, this stage is also marked by a growing federal presence in managed-care regulation.

Mandates on the Standard of Care

A controversial new breed of statute mandates benefits and sets medical policies for health plans. In essence, they create standards of care by legislation that reflect a growing consensus that managed care's emphasis on cost containment has pushed the standard of care in a direction thought to be too parsimonious. Perhaps above all, these statutes reflect a concern that plan administrators, rather than physicians, are making medical decisions.

Maternity length-of-stay bills may be the most publicized of this type of regulation. Departing from its traditional hands-off approach to managed-care regulation, Congress passed the Newborns' and Mothers' Health Protection Act of 1996, requiring ERISA plans to allow a forty-eight-hour hospital stay for normal deliveries.[5] At least forty states have passed similar statutes or variations thereof. Two states, Iowa and Maine, require adherence to American College of Obstetricians and Gynecologists (ACOG) guidelines rather than mandating specific lengths of stay (Kertesz 1996).

Legislation of this type often misses the mark. For example, bone marrow transplantation is not medically indicated for many breast cancer patients, yet Minnesota law requires that bone marrow transplantation be available to all breast cancer patients (Minn. Stat. Ann. sec. 62A.309 (West 1996)). Similarly, legislation mandating specific lengths of stay for a mastectomy ignores the fact that the term *mastectomy* describes a wide range of procedures with differing needs for hospitalization.

The approach taken by Iowa and Maine demonstrates a moderation in this standard-of-care legislative trend. The role of the physician, albeit with the standardizing influence of practice guidelines, may be put back into the treatment decision. States then set boundaries, not prescribe treatment. This approach also allows for changes in the standard of care due to medical advances. Such flexibility, or responsiveness, is often lacking in regulatory structures.

Access to Care

The issue of direct access is of increased interest to state legislatures. In response to aggressive denials of payment by health plans for emergency room treatment, many states have taken up measures to provide direct access to coverage for emergency room screenings. At least sixteen states have passed standards requiring insurers and managed care organizations (MCOs) to pay for emergency screenings if a prudent layperson would believe that such care was necessary (Laudicina et al. 1998). "Direct access" statutes also permit healthcare plan members to bypass the primary care physician and go directly to a specialist without a referral. The vast majority of states now require managed-care organizations to allow women to bypass the primary care physician for certain obstetrics or gynecology care.

Other access statutes vary widely as to the conditions covered or the type of specialist to whom direct access is granted. It is not clear why one state may mandate access to dermatologists (Fla.), while another mandates access to doctors of oriental medicine (N.M.). Similarly, a small number of states have begun mandating coverage for individual disorders, for example, growth cell stimulating factor injections; prostate screening; and treatment for phenylketonuria (PKU).

Gag Clauses

A strong movement is afoot at both the state and federal level to prohibit so-called gag clauses from managed-care contracts with physicians. Such clauses seek to restrict physicians from discussing all appropriate medical options with their patients, particularly those not covered by the health plan. Most states now ban such clauses, and, according to HCFA, gag clauses in Medicare and Medicaid contracts are a violation of federal law (Bureau of National Affairs 1996b). Also, at least one court has held that a gag policy by a health plan may constitute a breach of a fiduciary duty under ERISA (*Weiss v. Cigna Healthcare, Inc*, 972 F.Supp. 748, 750 (S.D. N.Y. 1997)).

Meanwhile, a study by the U.S. General Accounting Office (GAO) (1997) demonstrates that gag clauses are disappearing from provider contracts. However, this report points to an even more significant barrier to physician-patient communication that may be much more difficult to eliminate. The physician-HMO contractual relationship itself may make physicians feel constrained to limit communication with patients. The growing economic dependence of physicians on managed care is enhanced by the short duration (typically one year) of the terms of most provider-HMO contracts and the use of "without cause" termination clauses.[6]

Physician Deselection

Many now see that the emphasis has shifted from AWP laws that mandate the "selection" of physicians to the more narrow issue of "deselection," as part of a growing concern with patient and physician due process rights (Miller 1997; Laudicina et al. 1998; Bureau of National Affairs 1996c). This emphasis fits within the pattern of patient access laws now favored by states. In general, states are beginning to regulate the provider relationship with the managed-care organization by requiring provider access to information about standards for acceptance into a network, reasons for termination, and access to economic profiles of physicians' practice patterns (Miller 1997; Terry 1998). However, even the states most active on this issue have not addressed the continuity and access hurdles created by industry-wide contracts that are renewable annually. Only Maine requires reasons for nonrenewals and the opportunity for physicians to appeal (1997 Me. Laws 163, section 2, not applicable to cases involving "imminent harm to patient care") (see also Terry 1998).

Hand in hand with restraints on deselection, some states now require that for certain conditions physicians must continue to be paid for treatment rendered even after termination of the contract with the managed-care organization (Families USA 1998). Typically, such continuances may range from 60 to 120 days and cover a variety of medical conditions. However, with the exception of third trimester pregnancy and a limited number of acute conditions, such protections will only provide a brief transition period for most patients with more chronic conditions.

While less than satisfying, this stage of regulation is generally regarded as an improvement over the blunt anti-managed-care approach of a few years earlier. Legislatures became more active in addressing consumer concerns, particularly those related to access and quality. Certain measures adopted during this period, such as emergency room access, broad access to obstetrics and gynecology services, and some limited post-termination care, may continue to be part of the menu of managed-care reforms. This notwithstanding, we note the following problems.

First, the regulatory initiatives are targeted too narrowly. Measures mandating standards of care or access to seemingly randomly selected specialists may peel away specific anticonsumer practices, but they ignore the far greater number of quality and access concerns of consumers who lack lobbying clout or a sympathetic media. Ironically, drive-through deliveries and mastectomies received so much negative publicity that they disappeared from many health plans even before mandatory length-of-stay statutes were in place (Moran 1997).

Second, they ignore more deeply rooted barriers to improved quality and access. Generally speaking, the statutes adopted attempt to address consumer disquiet over the shift in the locus of medical decision making in managed care. To a certain extent outlawing gag clauses and adopting due process standards for physician deselection address such concerns. However, broader-based requirements, such as requiring a physician to oversee the development of medical policies and practices of the organization and holding health plans liable for medical decisions through tort law, may provide an incentive for medical decision making that will enhance the access to and quality of care for the benefit of all plan members. Similarly, outlawing gag clauses, which have largely disappeared from provider contracts, does not ensure free communication between patient and doctor or enhance patient access to medically necessary care as long as more pervasive industry practices are left unchecked. Physician economic reliance on managed care, the nature of managed-care provider contracts, and physician incentive plans may infringe these communications to a far greater extent.

Third, mandating standards is a particularly troubling development. The embrace of this approach, especially for obstetrics, has created second thoughts. It is better in the long run, for both quality and cost, to manage care through the creation of guidelines, where feasible, but to leave individual decisions up to individual doctors and patients.

It is submitted that with the fourth stage of managed-care regulation we may be entering a more mature phase.

The Fourth Stage: Toward a Regulatory Middle Ground

New approaches to managed-care regulation are being advanced that seem to be carving out a middle ground between the consumer backlash and the market forces approaches. We submit that regulation in each of the areas discussed in the following sections contains more uniform, flexible, and nuanced regulatory structures, which bring managed-care regulation closer to its objectives of promoting quality, access, and cost containment.

Regulation of Risk-Bearing Provider Groups

As managed care evolves, perhaps the most significant new development is that of the risk-bearing provider group (RBPG) (Overbey and Hall 1996). RBPGs take a variety of forms, including integrated delivery systems (IDSs), independent practice associations (IPAs), physician hospital organizations (PHOs), and provider sponsored organizations (PSOs), which lead to a welter of acronyms (Burns and Thorpe 1993). As Robinson points out, as managed-care organizations reinvent themselves, they seem to be abandoning the traditional vertically integrated staff or group model for "virtual integration" (1996). Rather than the unified ownership and employed physicians that characterize vertical integration, virtual integration entails contractual relationships between health plans and integrated medical groups or independent practice associations. Under virtual integration, the physicians, rather than the HMO or the hospital, bear much of the financial risk of managed care. Also, a growing number of hospital and physician groups are bypassing the health plan and seeking to contract directly with employers for their services on a risk-bearing basis.

Physician members of these new organizations share in the financial risk of treating patients, yet they are only beginning to be regulated in any significant fashion. Although regulators in most states claim that fully capitated RBPGs are subject to state licensure under HMO licensure laws, in reality very few, if any, appear to be licensed (Kaufman and Webster 1995). Only a few states have developed laws specific to provider-sponsored organizations. This may be due, in part, to state concerns of ERISA preemption. Minnesota, for example, has addressed this development by adapting its HMO licensure to authorize the establishment of community integrated service networks (CISNs). CISNs are licensed by the insurance commissioner to provide health services to 50,000 or fewer enrollees. CISNs must maintain a minimum net worth of at least $1 million. The same minimum threshold applies to HMOs, but CISNs have a three-year phase-in to meet the net worth requirement (see Minnesota Integrated Services Network Act, Minn. Stat. Ann. sec. 62N.309 (West 1997)).

Regulation of RBPGs is controversial. The NAIC characterizes RBPGs as "in the business of insurance" and argues that they should comply with state solvency and consumer protection regulations (NAIC 1996b). The NAIC's definition of "business of insurance" would include capitated payments as well as risk corridors, withholds, or pooling arrangements.[7] Opponents of the NAIC's position on the regulation of RBPGs argue that providers who contract directly with employers only assume the limited risk for the specific services they agree to provide. If made to comply with insurance regulations, RBPGs would be shut out of the market entirely, and competition, as well as innovation, would be stifled.

While we leave an in-depth examination of these emerging entities and market dynamics to others (e.g., Berenson 1997; Gabel 1997; Robinson 1996; Shortell 1994, 1996), we realize that the market will likely play a significant role in the viability of these emerging RBPGs. Therefore, regulation that can adapt to these entities, such as the Minnesota CISN approach, may provide a safety net that promotes quality as it protects the fiscal integrity of these organizations as they compete in the marketplace.

At the federal level, under the Balanced Budget Act of 1997 (BBA) (Pub. Law 105–33 section 1851 (a)(2)(A), 1855 (d)), PSOs may contract directly with Medicare to provide services. Solvency requirements have been developed for these PSOs through a process of negotiated rule making (63 Fed. Reg. 25360, et seq.), whereby a committee of representatives of stakeholders was convened. The committee included representatives of the insurance industry, consumer groups, and provider and medical associations. As discussed further in a later section, this ability to draw experts from across the country, which is generally unique to the federal system, provides an opportunity to learn about the issues confronting the entities to be regulated, allowing for "responsive" regulatory oversight. States may find such rules an important starting point for their own requirements. Also, organizations such as the NAIC may allow greater communication among states and thereby broaden the forum for debate.

Disclosing and Regulating Provider Incentives

In 1998 we saw some evidence of new methods of regulation that may define the oversight of the future. Perhaps the most thoughtful contribution was that of HCFA. HCFA has had legislative responsibility for regulating physician incentive plans (PIPs) since the passage of the Omnibus Reconciliation Act of 1990 (OBRA) (Pub. Law No. 101–508, 104 Stat. 1388, codified at 42 U.S.C. section 1395mm (1998) (Medicare); *ibid.* section 4731, codified at 42 U.S.C. section 1396 (m)(1998) (Medicaid)). This legislation required that any physician incentive plan, defined as "any compensation arrangement between a managed-care organization and a physician or physician group that may directly or indirectly have the effect of reducing or eliminating service furnished to Medicare beneficiaries or Medicaid recipients enrolled in managed-care organizations," be the subject of rules promulgated by HCFA (42 U.S.C. section 1395mm (1998)).

In general, the PIP rules (see Fed. Reg. 69,035 (1996)) now require plans that place providers at substantial financial risk for referral services (SFRFRS) to meet stop-loss insurance requirements, to comply with patient survey requirements, to disclose physicians' incentive plans to HCFA and upon request to patients, and to survey patients.[8] Substantial financial risk is defined as 25 percent of potential payments for covered services. Large plans (25,000 patients) are not considered at substantial financial risk because the risk is spread over a large number of patients.

The greatest problems with managed care are likely to occur in the cost-quality trade-offs that result from placing physicians at risk for providing further care. HCFA's approach to balancing these trade-offs has much to emulate. First, the disclosure requirements recognize the importance of monitoring the risk for both managed-care organizations and physician groups and of maintaining actuarially adequate pools of patients. Second, it is innovative. The use of patient surveys, a requirement for stop-loss insurance, and encouragement of disclosures are evidence of a more mature stage of regulation of managed care.

Requiring full disclosure of risk-sharing arrangements enables a regulatory agency to target its oversight. The disclosure requirements apply to *all* Medicare and Medicaid contracting health plans, allowing for broader comparisons. Moreover, the regulations require that, when there is more than one level of contracting, the financial arrangement that is to be reported is the tier under which the treating physician is operating. A summary of the PIP must be provided to enrollees upon request.

The use of patient surveys to understand how patients perceive the care they are receiving is an exciting development. To get a complete picture of patient opinion, plans must survey current enrollees and disenrollees. Regulation that enables consumers to give voice to their complaints may be a potent force in prompting the organization to remedy situations giving rise to such complaints (Rodwin 1996). To maximize the usefulness of surveys, careful coordination with other information collection strategies should be carried out. Mandating the use of surveys developed by the Agency for Health (Care) Policy and Research (AHCPR) for both Medicare and Medicaid as part of the

Consumer Assessment of Health Plans Study (CAHPS) would allow for more productive comparisons of data.

Using other developing quality measures in a similar fashion would allow full evaluation of the cost-quality trade-offs. For example, the government could require that there be much more specific attention to monitoring adverse events, compliance with Health Plan Employer Data and Information Set (HEDIS) quality criteria, and to specific outcome measures in those areas in which physicians are being placed at greater risk.

It is likely that permutations of this approach will be much more effective than are many of the forms of oversight that the states are now pursuing. State legislation in this area tends to be vague, prohibiting plans from using financial incentives that will directly or indirectly induce physicians to limit medically necessary care, and provides uneven case-by-case enforcement mechanisms.

Changing Interpretations of ERISA Preemption

Our earlier discussion of federal preemption of AWP laws notwithstanding, ERISA case law following *Travelers* and *DeBuono* demonstrates a shift toward a more narrow view of ERISA preemption of state law. While many of the cases cited here and in the following section were decided during earlier "stages," the significance of these various strains of interpretation will likely coalesce and begin to be felt during this stage.

Recent jurisprudence suggests that states may be able to avoid ERISA pre-emption by innovative interpretation of their own law. In *Napoletano v. Cigna Healthcare of Conn.* (680 A.2d 127 (Conn. 1996), cert. denied, 117 S. Ct. 1106 (1996)), claims centered on alleged misrepresentations made by the plan as to the status of the physicians as members of Cigna's provider network and their eligibility for membership in the network. The court held that such claims brought under the state unfair trade practices and unfair insurance practices act, the managed-care act, and common law did not "relate to" an employee plan but sought to have the defendant enforce the plan it had chosen to create and administer. Significantly, the court acknowledged that it would apply an admittedly narrow test for ERISA preemption, limiting preemption to state action that *demonstrably burdens* ERISA plans (680 A. 2d at 140). Holdings such as this may encourage Connecticut and other states to further regulate managed care. However, the breadth of state jurisdiction in these matters, given ERISA, is still very uncertain.

Perhaps mindful of ERISA's "vacuum," federal courts are beginning to interpret the ERISA statute itself as entailing protection for consumers. In the case of *Shea v. Esensten* (107 F.3d 625 (8th Cir. 1997), cert. denied, 118 S. Ct. 297 (1997)), the court held that financial incentives that discourage a treating doctor from providing essential health care referrals for conditions covered under the plan must be disclosed and the failure to do so is a breach of ERISA's fiduciary duties[9] (see also *Drolet v. Healthsource, Inc.*, 968 F. Supp. 757 (N.H.

1997)). The United States Court of Appeals for the Seventh Circuit attempted to take *Shea* a step further, holding that when physicians own and control the health plan an incentive structure that influences physicians to withhold care to save money *for themselves* may rise to the level of a breach of the ERISA fiduciary duty (*Herdrich v. Pegram*, 154 F.3d 362 (7th Cir. 1998), reversed by 120 S. Ct. 2143 (2000)). As noted earlier, *Weiss v. Cigna Healthcare, Inc.*, held that a gag clause may violate the plan's fiduciary duty.

Federal courts have generally been unwilling to make such a substantive interpretation of a relatively thin regulation existing under ERISA. These cases likely indicate more willingness to engage in reasonable federal oversight of managed care on the part of the federal court, and in this roundabout and limited way they may accomplish some state consumer protection goals.[10]

Perhaps the most controversial aspect of ERISA preemption is its impact on managed-care tort liability. We address this issue in the next section.

Managed-Care Liability

Both ERISA preemption and certain state laws have served to immunize managed-care organizations from tort liability. Recently, however, these barriers to liability have shown signs of weakening.

A number of court decisions, most notably, *Corcoran v. United Health Care, Inc.* (965 F.2d 1321 (5th Cir. 1992), cert. denied, 113 S. Ct. 812 (1992)),[11] have held that compensation under state law for injuries resulting from health plan negligence is preempted by ERISA. The civil enforcement scheme set out in section 502(a) of ERISA allows only for reimbursement of benefits promised and not received. Thus the Corcorans were left without a remedy for the allegedly negligent utilization review decision that resulted in the death of their unborn child. However, courts now seem less willing to interpret ERISA as insulating managed-care organizations from liability for negligence.

The influential case of *Dukes v. U.S. Healthcare, Inc.* (57 F.3d 250 (3d Cir. 1995), cert. denied, 116 S. Ct. 564 (1995))[12] presented a new way to look at such cases. Where claims of plan negligence are raised, the court must distinguish between claims that focus on the "quality" of medical benefits received and those that concern the "quantity" of benefits received. The latter is completely preempted, but with regard to the former, the Dukes' court stated that because ERISA is silent, complete preemption cannot be found.

This *Dukes* quality-quantity distinction was applied in the case of *Pappas v. Asbel* (724 A.2d 889 (Pa. 1999), vacated and remanded subnom., 120 S. Ct. 2686 (2000)), and the court rejected an ERISA preemption argument. In that case the plaintiff was allegedly injured as a result of the HMO's cost-conscious delay in authorizing emergency room personnel to transfer the plaintiff to a facility equipped to treat the plaintiff's condition. The district court pointed out that ERISA was enacted prior to the invention of the cost containment system utilized in the review at issue and concluded that Congress could not have intended to foreclose recovery to plan beneficiaries injured by negligent medical decisions based on cost containment rationale.[13] In general, courts are split as to whether the *Dukes* or *Corcoran* rationale applies.

The breadth of ERISA preemption is being further tested as states pass statutes permitting suits against managed-care plans. In many states the "corporate practice of medicine" doctrine may work to shield managed-care organizations from such liability (Butler 1997). Under this doctrine, because health plans cannot practice medicine, they cannot be held liable for negligent medical decisions. However, recent legislation, most notably in Texas and Missouri, has been enacted to abrogate that doctrine (see Texas Health Care Liability Act, Tex. Civ. Prac. & Rem. Code Ann. Sections 88.001–88.003 (West 1998); Mo. H.B. 335, repealing Rev. St. Mo. Section 345.505.3, adding section 345.627).

The Missouri statute simply removes the barrier to suits, leaving it to the courts to determine the type of lawsuits that can be brought and the standard of care required. The Texas statute takes an additional step in creating a new cause of action where a plan fails to use "ordinary care" in denying or delaying payment for care recommended by a physician or other provider.[14] The law appears to make health plans liable for their own "health care treatment decisions," as well as for actions by employees and agents who make coverage decisions or directly deliver care (section 88002(B)). Prior to bringing a lawsuit, the enrollee is required to exhaust the appeal remedy (external to the plan) established by the statute.

The case of *Corporate Health Insurance v. Texas Department of Insurance* (12 F. Supp.2d 597 (S.D. Tex. 1998, affd in part and reversed in part, 215 F. 3d 526 (5th Cir. 2000) petn. for cert. filed, 69 USLW 3317 (10/24/2000)) involved an ERISA preemption challenge to the new Texas statute. While an analysis of the opinion is beyond our scope, it upheld those aspects of the statute that permit a cause of action against managed-care plans.[15] The court noted that such actions would be evaluated on a case-by-case basis. Those claims based upon the *Dukes* quality of care rationale are not preempted, while those claims asserting negligent denial of medically necessary benefits, such as in *Corcoran*, are preempted. Whether such a distinction is workable will be established by subsequent cases. However, redress by the statute in some cases may well be stymied by ERISA preemption.

An increasing number of states are considering similar legislation (Laudicina et al. 1998, vii). Moreover, not all states bar suits against managed-care plans, nor, as noted earlier, is preemption always an insurmountable hurdle to suit in the ERISA context. For example, a recent Pennsylvania appeals court case recognized a cause of action for corporate negligence against an HMO for allegedly negligent advice given to the enrollee through the HMO's emergency medical advice line *(Shannon v. HealthAmerica, 718 A.2d 828 (Pa. Super. 1998))*.

Acknowledging that medical decisions are made by managed-care organizations, physician licensure boards in some states are applying greater scrutiny to coverage decisions made by medical directors of managed-care organizations (see *Murphy v. Board of Medical Examiners of Arizona,* 949 P.2d 530 (1997)). The Maryland Board of Physician Quality Assurance is presently contemplating specific regulations allowing that body to take actions against medical directors (Page 1998).

Given the breadth of ERISA preemption, what really matters, of course, is how this debate is resolved at the federal level. The controversial role of Congress and the proposals under consideration are discussed in the next section.

Current Legislative Action on the Federal Level

Over the past two years, widespread support for federal managed-care legislation has been in evidence. The health-care Consumer Bill of Rights was developed by the President's Advisory Commission on Consumer Protection and Quality in the Health Care Industry and is viewed by many as a blueprint for needed reform. A number of bills sponsored by both political parties, by public and private sectors, and by those inside and outside of managed care have been introduced. However, despite predictions that managed-care legislation would be enacted by Congress in 1998, preoccupation with the presidential impeachment and the events leading up to it precluded their fulfillment. Moreover, some interpret the mid-term election results as falling short of a voter mandate for broad federal reform (Nather 1998).

Bills have been offered by both the Republican and Democratic leadership—the House Republican Patient Protection Act (H.R. 4250), was introduced in the 106th Congress, and the Democratic Patients' Bill of Rights Act (S. 6), which has recently been reintroduced. Prospects of either being passed are uncertain.[16] A description of these bills is beyond our scope. However, the bills introduced in the 106th Congress demonstrated basic differences of opinion as to what role the federal government should play in regulating managed care. The Patients' Bill of Rights Act contained wide-ranging consumer protections and would amend ERISA to allow for negligence actions against managed-care plans. The Patient Protection Act was more narrowly drawn and did not provide for suits against managed-care plans. Thus, how and how far governmental activism in the regulation of managed care will proceed at the federal level remains to be seen.[17]

Interestingly, the presidential commission deadlocked on just these issues (Pear 1998). Consumer advocates, doctors, and some labor leaders on the commission favored recommending a federal enforcement mechanism of the Bill of Rights. Commissioners from insurance companies, managed-care organizations, and businesses opposed increased industry regulation and argued that voluntary compliance would accomplish the same result. Not surprising, the Commission was similarly split over the right of enrollees to compensation for injuries due to improper denial of benefits.

As noted throughout our discussion, this fourth stage of regulation has shown potential to increase quality and access while balancing costs by overseeing physician incentives and by moving toward the adoption of tort-based incentives for managed care. Efforts are also afoot to promote quality by protecting the fiscal integrity of organizations, especially emerging entities. However, recent reports of rising managed-care costs—and premiums—may lead to a reexamination of certain cost-quality trade-offs and may limit the number and types of reforms that succeed (Kilborn 1998). Efforts to extend liability to managed-care organizations and the trend to broaden provider panels may be closely examined by states and health plans. State activism during this stage seems likely, as there was legislation introduced in every state in 1999 and 2000.

Discussion and Recommendations

Broader-based regulatory structures that avoid mandating standards of medical care hold more promise for accomplishing the objectives of managed-care regulation. The question is, what particular regulatory structures seem the most promising? From the legislative and regulatory initiatives we have reviewed, we note six regulatory approaches that demonstrate particular promise in reaching these goals society has set for managed care.

Setting a Federal Floor

Although the issue of legal enforceability of the Consumer Bill of Rights and Responsibilities was hotly debated and failed to produce a consensus, we believe that an enforcement mechanism is needed, given the rapid evolution of health care and the risk of inattention to matters of quality. The significant level of state legislative activity in this area, and its gaps in areas of quality assurance, supports our proposal. To this end we recommend that a set of minimum requirements be set at the federal level to be administered by the states. The task of enforcement is simply too large an undertaking for the federal government. States are much better positioned to enforce the minimum requirements and possess the expertise to tailor regulation to the concerns of their populations and to the specifics of their health-care organizations. To permit states to experiment, ERISA should be amended to remove the preemption barrier to state regulation. The federal-state division of labor will thus be better defined, but with opportunity for collaboration.

In general, the federal floor should be comprised of those elements on the regulatory menu that society has appeared to decide by consensus should be included in managed-care regulation. Broadly stated, the floor should require disclosure of information to consumers; choice of providers and plans; access to care, including a prudent layperson standard for emergency room services; reasonable access to specialists; some safeguards for those in need of continuity of care following physician terminations for reasons other than quality; a gag clause ban; informed consent; patient confidentiality protections; nondiscrimination against enrollees; grievance and appeals procedures; and quality assurance mechanisms.

Again, we recommend against those elements from this menu that mandate standards of care or seek to appease random interests. Once the federal floor is established, states would remain free to require more of health plans.

Meaningful and Standardized Reporting Requirements

As the HCFA PIP reporting requirements demonstrate, the collection of data from plans and patients provides an important opportunity to learn about the regulated entities and about the effect the regulations may be having, both positive and negative. The Democrat-sponsored Patients' Bill of Rights Act appropriately encourages uniform reporting. Under section 112 of the act health plans must collect uniform quality data that include a "minimum uniform data set" and report such data in a standardized format to the secretary. This data set includes aggregate utilization data, the demographic characteristics of members, disease-specific and age-specific mortality rates, satisfaction of enrollees (including data on voluntary disenrollment and grievance and appeals data), and quality indicators.

More specific measures should not be overlooked. Readmissions, rates of complications, as well as consumer complaints provide important information on quality. The challenge of quality regulation is to keep pace with developments in the science of quality measurements so that regulations dovetail with quality tools as they are developed. Others have documented the potential for quality measures, as well as the difficulty in arriving at them (Gosfield 1997; Cleary and Edgman-Levitan 1997; Brook 1997). One potentially powerful tool for translating developments in this area into more effective regulations is the establishment of a federal quality commission, such as that proposed by the Patients' Bill of Rights Act.

A Federal Quality Commission

The rapidly changing area of health-care quality and its measurement is ideally suited to the employment of a federally based commission. Some versions of proposed patients' bill of rights legislation would establish such a commission. This approach is not new. The Balanced Budget Act of 1997 established the

Medicare Payment Advisory Commission (MPAC), whose membership includes prominent experts in a variety of relevant fields. MPAC brings its considerable expertise to bear in weighing the implications of policy change across the many components of the Medicare program, working toward consistency in the policies it recommends.

As with MPAC, a Federal Quality Commission would be free to consider short-term as well as long-term implications of existing policy and regulation, an important function given the often politically charged topics for which its advice is sought. The continuing evaluation and input of the commission should increase the likelihood that regulation will innovate rather than stagnate when addressing the complex area of health-care quality.

Given a regulatory structure with a federal floor, states are able to benefit from the commission's work. However, it is incumbent on state regulators to voluntarily communicate with their counterparts in other states to share information so as to maximize the quality of its health-care institutions. Involvement of nongovernmental organizations, such as medical societies and the NAIC, in the exchange of information should also be encouraged.

Understandable and Uniform Enrollee Disclosure Information

Many states and proposed patients' bill of rights legislation list information that must be disclosed to participants and beneficiaries at the time of initial coverage under the plan. To maximize the usefulness of this information, however, it should be made available to potential enrollees who are in the process of choosing a health plan. A uniform and understandable method of providing this information will enhance the ability of the consumer to make an informed choice at that more critical juncture.

The scope of the information provided says much about the perceived role of the consumer in making choices about health-care coverage. In addition to the "nuts and bolts" of accessing health care (obtaining referrals, prior authorizations, grievance procedures, etc.), an informed consumer also needs to know what financial incentives are offered providers and what quality data are available. Making information available to patients about cost containment strategies, as the new HCFA regulations and some of the proposed bills require, is an important step in involving patients more directly in decisions about their health care. Such measures could also play a role in restoring consumer trust in managed care.

Researchers are beginning to measure consumer interest and understanding of quality data (Cleary et al. 1997; Schneider and Epstein 1998). Until we know more, common sense and the strong tradition of informed consent tell us to provide uniform and understandable information. However, there are some limits on disclosure. In fact, we would argue that when raw information disseminated to patients is beyond their expertise to interpret, or is prone to misinterpretation, because regulators, politicians, or providers themselves cannot agree on what impact it should have on health-care decisions, this amounts to a regulatory cop-out.

For example, one version of a patients' bill of rights provides that enrollees be informed of the plan's medical loss ratio (MLR). The MLR is the statistic that measures the percent of managed-care premium revenue that is spent on medical care, as distinct from administration and profit. Despite significant public interest in this statistic, critics question its value as an indicator of managed-care quality or efficiency (Robinson 1998).

According to Robinson, the MLR is a poor indicator of both quality of care and administrative waste. For example, we do know that physician choice is a key ingredient of patient satisfaction. Staff model HMOs that provide the least provider choice typically have lower administrative expenses. Conversely, those plans that provide the most choice are those with higher administrative expenses.

Further undermining the reliability of the MLR is a lack of standardized accounting practices in arriving at the ratio. According to a study by Turnbull and Kane, nearly one-third of the difference in MLR values reported by HMOs could be attributable to accounting differences (1998). The authors argue convincingly that if greater significance is attributed to MLRs, there will be increased incentive to employ whatever accounting strategies will create the most favorable MLR. Thus, supplying this particular raw statistic would constitute a regulatory cop-out. The Joint Commission on the Accreditation of Healthcare Organizations (JCAHO) is widely recognized as an inspector of quality in hospital care. By contrast to the MLR, when the JCAHO team completes an inspection, the team does not simply post scores but translates its inspection results into meaningful information to guide the health-care facility in improving quality. The concept of "responsive regulation" posits regulation as a learning experience.

However, even mandating the disclosure of meaningful and easily interpreted information may constitute a regulatory cop-out. Merely publishing quality data does not prevent low-scoring health plans from remaining in business (Epstein 1998). Because most private purchasers choose health plans based on cost and size, not quality, and most consumers are limited to health plans selected by their employers, receiving information that a plan has a poor quality rating is not helpful. Thus, in the absence of market incentives to select for quality, alert and responsive regulation should go beyond disclosure and set a tolerance level for health plan quality. Barring new enrollees from joining health plans below the tenth percentile of the industry may not only spare potential enrollees from substandard care but may succeed in raising the standards of the industry.

Managed-Care Accountability

The debate over managed-care liability echoes the long-standing question of cost-quality trade-offs under managed care. The extension of tort liability to managed-care plans is a positive step toward addressing the need for an analytical framework for ascribing liability given the industry's influence on treatment decisions. Individuals within managed care that make "medical" decisions may be less likely to err on the side of cost over quality if personal liability in tort or disciplinary action may result from such decisions. Liability may also reduce consumer perception that coverage denials are often arbitrary and unfair (Butler 1997).

Although medical malpractice, in general, is not regarded as a significant factor in deterring substandard medical care by individual physicians, empirical research has demonstrated that its deterrence signal is felt at the organizational level (Brennan 1995). As the organizational structure becomes more important, as in the managed-care setting, the threat of malpractice liability to the organization will more likely be translated into greater concern for quality of care (Abraham and Weiler 1994; Studdert and Brennan 1997). Thus theories of no-fault and enterprise liability are particularly suited to the managed-care organization. By focusing the organization on prevention, this type of liability would bring about greater deterrence of medical injury than does the present system, especially if experience rating is employed (Studdert and Brennan 1997; Brennan and Berwick 1996).

The extension of malpractice liability to the managed-care organization will most likely require the amending of ERISA. We encourage such an amendment.

Encouragement of Innovation

An area of promising regulation is the development of short-term projects for pilot testing new regulatory mechanisms. An example of a regulatory mechanism suitable for such testing is the "ombudsperson" concept contained in a number of regulatory initiatives at both the state and federal level. One version of a proposed Patients' Bill of Rights defines the function of an ombudsperson as "to provide counseling and assistance to enrollees dissatisfied with their treatment by health insurance issuers and group health plans in regard to such coverage or plans and with respect to grievances and appeals regarding determinations under such coverage or plans."

The ombudsperson represents a new approach to addressing patient grievances and lends itself to experimentation in a small number of states. If certain benchmarks of consumer, provider, and health plan satisfaction are met on an experimental basis, broader use would be indicated. The opportunity for smaller-scale experimentation would also encourage innovation.

Pilot testing is not feasible for all circumstances. However, responsive regulation is always testing methods of regulation. Regulators should evaluate the effectiveness of such mechanisms on the quality, access, and cost, as well as their success in encouraging innovation. Where possible, this should be done on an iterative basis.

Conclusion

As the regulation of managed care proceeds, we can only hope that there will be continued focus on more nuanced approaches to regulations. Throughout the foregoing, we have described what we believe to be important factors in creating regulatory structures that will meet the traditional objectives of regulation while not discouraging the influence of market forces in helping to achieve these same objectives. After all, managed care may only be the start of a more effective health-care market (Drake 1997).

Regulation should acknowledge that quality, not managed care itself, is the problem. Thus, we should move beyond reflexive anti-managed-care legislation. Utilization and quality review may provide some improvement, especially as the development of quality indicators continues to mature. We need to acknowledge that managed-care organizations make medical decisions and that holding them accountable may enhance quality and patient trust in the system. The goal of maintaining consumer trust in the doctor-patient relationship, as well as in the triangular relationship of doctor-patient-plan, remains vital.

A greater understanding of the impact of physician economic dependence on managed care organizations is needed. Also needed is a federal and state division of labor that plays to the strength of each while promoting collaboration. A continued ERISA vacuum may thwart state and federal regulators in assuming such optimal roles.

Despite hurdles, regulators should continue to embrace better rules that seek to infuse a collaborative sensibility, a mutual learning experience, into the relationship between the regulator and the regulated. Working together, emphasizing the critical element, that is, physician risk, and applying techniques of quality measurement and quality improvement would seem to be our best bet to assure patient safety and to help doctors ethically care for patients.

NOTES

1. A typical grievance procedure law requires plans to inform enrollees of grievance procedures, remind them of it at the time of denial, and set deadlines for resolving grievances, depending on the medical urgency (Page 1996).

2. NCQA is an independent, nonprofit organization that assesses, measures, and reports on the quality of care provided by managed-care organizations. NCQA's standards focus on six fundamental areas: utilization management; credentialing; quality management and improvement; members' rights and responsibilities; preventive health services; and medical records. See chapter 10.

3. See also *Blue Cross and Blue Shield of Alabama v. Neilsen,* 917 F.Supp. 1532 (N.D. Ala. 1996). affd. in part, vacated in part, and remanded, 142 F.3d 1375 (11th Cir. 1998). Eds. note: as a result of the Eleventh Circuit opinion, the ERISA issue was mooted.

4. At least one court has relied on the *Travelers* and *DeBuono* cases to conclude that an AWP statute does not "relate to" ERISA plans and is not preempted by ERISA, *American Drug Stores, Inc. v. Harvard Pilgrim Health Care, Inc.,* 973 F.Supp. 60 (D.C. Mass. 1997).

5. ERISA has also been amended to allow for parity for mental health coverage, 29 U.S.C. section 1185a. See Mental Health Parity Act of 1996, 42 U.S.C. 30088–5.

6. Nearly all of the contracts surveyed by the GAO (1997) were for a one-year period, renewable for a one-year period. Seventy-two percent of the contracts surveyed contained an "at will" or "without cause" termination clause.

7. In capitation the provider accepts a set per patient fee regardless of the amount of services that the patient requires. The corridor of risk is the amount of risk assumed by the provider before a "stop loss" policy attachment point is reached. When withholds and risk pools are in place, the managed-care organization deducts a certain amount from each provider's payment and places the money in a pool to pay for costs of referrals that exceed the managed-care organization's budgeted amount. If the cost of services exceed the budget, the provider loses some or all of those funds. See NAIC 1996b, 17–18; see generally, Latham 1996.

8. See Dallek and Hasenberg 1997 for a description of the regulatory requirements.

9. Editors' note: In *Ehlmann v. Kaiser Foundation Health Plan of Texas,* 198 F.3d 552 (5th Cir. 2000), the court held that ERISA does not impose a fiduciary duty on health plans to disclose physician financial incentives to enrollees. The *Elmann* court distinguished *Shea v. Esensten* as a "special circumstances" case in which the patient had repeatedly requested that the incentivized physician refer him to a cardiologist.

10. Editors' note: Although the United States Supreme Court, in reversing the Seventh Circuit in *Herdrich,* found that ERISA fiduciary standards were not violated by the use of physician financial incentives, broad dicta in that opinion appears to open the door to greater oversight of managed-care organizations under traditional state laws. See *Pegram v. Herdrich,* 120 S.Ct. 2143 (2000). The Supreme Court also specifically left open the question of whether ERISA fiduciary standards imposed a duty to disclose the existence of physician financial incentives.

11. See also *Kuhl v. Lincoln National Health Plan,* 999 F.2d 298 (8th Cir. 1993) (ERISA preempted claim of negligent denial of precertification for surgery); *Elsesser v. Hospital College of Osteopathic Med.,* 802 F.Supp. 1286 (E.D. Pa. 1992) (claim against HMO for failure to fund the use of diagnostic medical device preempted by ERISA, but claim of HMO negligence in selection, retention, and evaluation of physician not preempted). Compare *Kearney v. U.S. Healthcare, Inc.,* 859 F.Supp. 182 (E.D. Pa. 1994) (holding that ERISA preempts the plaintiff's direct negligence claim against U.S. Healthcare but not its vicarious liability claim).

12. In that case claims of vicarious and direct negligence against an HMO were not

completely preempted by ERISA. The Supreme Court vacated for reconsideration in light of its decision in *Pegram vs. Heidrich.*

13. See also *Bauman v. U.S. Healthcare, Inc.* 193 F.3d 151 (3rd Cir. 1999), cert. denied, 120 S. Ct. 2687 (2000), (where a newborn died as a result of alleged failure to diagnose meningitis, the claim that health plan was negligent in structuring its plan to allow for only a twenty-four-hour maternity/newborn hospital stay was not completely preempted by ERISA); *Ouellete v. Christ Hospital,* 942 F.Supp. 1160 (S.D. Oh. 1996) (in which a malpractice claim that an HMO breached its duty to the beneficiary by limiting hospital stays, and by enforcing such limits through unreasonable financial incentives with hospitals, was not completely preempted under ERISA). Both cases were removed to state court to determine ERISA conflict preemption. Along with *Pappas, Bauman* and *Ouellete* raise the question of the extent to which a health plan's causing its providers to act negligently toward beneficiaries overcomes the hurdle of ERISA preemption, making way for the beneficiary's common law cause of action.

14. For contrary holdings, see *Jass v. Prudential Health Care Plan, Inc.,* 88 F.3d 1482 (7th Cir. 1996) (ERISA completely preempts a malpractice claim on negligent utilization review); *Lancaster v. Kaiser Foundation Health Plan of Mid-Atlantic States, Inc.,* 958 F.Supp. 1137, 1147 (E.D. Va. 1997) (despite the allegation that health plan guidelines and cost standards prevented a complete assessment of the plaintiff's medical condition and proper and timely diagnosis, complete preemption under section 502 (a) was found because the claim "challenged an administrative decision that has the effect of denying benefits").

15. The court also held that ERISA preempted three statutory provisions that have been implemented by a number of states: a provision mandating an external review process, section 88.0003; a prohibition of the use of "hold harmless" clauses in provider contracts, section 88.002(g); and an anti–gag clause provision, section 88.002(f). Editors' note: The United States Court of Appeals for the Fifth Circuit later reversed the holding that ERISA preempted the hold harmless and anti-gag clause provisions.

16. Editor's note: On February 6, 2001, federal legislators introduced "Bipartisan Patient Protection Act(s)." Senators John McCain, R-AZ, John Edwards, D-NC, Edward Kennedy, D-MA, Lincoln Chafee, R-RI, Tom Harkin, D-IA, and Bob Graham, D-FL, introduced the Senate bills, and Reps. Greg Ganske, M.D., R-IA, and John Dingell, D-MI, introduced the House bills. Senator McCain stated that the proposed legislation would: give every American the right to choose his or her own doctor; cover all Americans with employer-based health insurance; ensure that all external reviews of medical decisions are conducted by independent and qualified physicians; and hold a health plan accountable when the plan makes a decision that harms or kills someone. The proposed law, as described by Senator McCain, would permit state-enacted patient protections; provide a federal cause of action for negligent plan administration (which will provide uniformity on how the health plans are administered); protect businesses from frivolous lawsuits; and hold insurers accountable for injuries arising from their actions. President George W. Bush, on the day after bipartisan patient rights legislation was introduced in the Senate and the House, issued a press release containing "Principles for a Bipartisan Patients' Bill of Rights." Bush's principles included the following: patient protections should apply to all Americans enrolled in health plans; a federal patients' rights law should provide rights such as access to emergency room and specialty care, direct access to certain doctors, access to needed prescription drugs and approved clinical trials, and a prohibition on "gag clauses"; patients should have a rapid

medical review process for denials of care; physicians should make medical decisions and patients should receive care in a timely manner; federal remedies should be expanded to hold health plans accountable for wrongful denial of care; and employers should be protected from frivolous or unnecessary lawsuits.

17. Editor's note: The 2001 Bipartisan Patient Protection Acts are pending as this book goes to press. References in the remainder of this chapter are to the earlier Republication Patient Protection Act and Democratic Patients' Bill of Rights.

REFERENCES

Abraham, K., and P. Weiler. 1994. "Enterprise Medical Liability and the Evolution of the American Health Care System." *Harvard Law Review* 108:381–436.

Advisory Commission on Consumer Protection and Quality in the Health Care Industry. 1998. *Quality First: Better Health Care for All Americans.* Washington, D.C.: U.S. Government Printing Office.

Berenson, R. 1997. "Beyond Competition." *Health Affairs* 16:171–80.

Blendon, R., et al. 1998. "Understanding the Managed Care Backlash." *Health Affairs* 17: 80–94.

Bodenheimer, T. 1997. "The HMO Backlash—Righteous or Reactionary?" *New Eng. J. Med.* 335:1601–3.

Brennan, T. 1995. "Letter: Questioning the Value of Liability in Medical Malpractice." *Health Affairs* 14:320–21.

Brennan, T., and D. Berwick. 1996. *New Rules: Regulation, Markets, and the Quality of American Health Care.* San Francisco, Calif.: Jossey-Bass.

Brook, R. 1997. "Managed Care Is Not the Problem, Quality Is." *JAMA* 278:1612–14.

Budetti, P. 1997. "Health Reform for the 21st Century?" *JAMA* 227:193.

Bureau of National Affairs. 1995. "State Law Consumer Protections Vary, May Leave Important Issues Unaddressed." *Health Law Reporter* 4:1841.

———. 1996a. "States Drop Comprehensive Reform, Take Up 'Anti-Managed Care' Efforts." *Health Law Reporter* 5:159.

———. 1996b. "Medicare." *Health Law Reporter* 5:1794.

———. 1996c. "As Action on 'Any Willing Provider' Laws Wanes, States Take up 'Direct Access' Bills." *Health Law Reporter* 6:390.

———. 1998. "Managed Care: State Legislation: Managed Care Bills Top State Agendas in 1999; Legislation Pending in Every State." *Health Law Reporter* 7:1996.

Burns, L., and D. Thorpe. 1993. "Trends and Models in Physician Hospital Organizations." *Health Care Management Review* 18:7.

Butler, P. 1997. *Managed Care Plan Liability: An Analysis of Texas and Missouri Legislation.* Menlo Park, Calif.: Kaiser Family Foundation.

Chassin, M., R. Galvin, and the National Roundtable on Health Care Quality, 1998. "The Urgent Need to Improve Health Care Quality." *JAMA* 280:1000–1005.

Chirba-Martin, M., and T. Brennan. 1994. "The Critical Role of ERISA in State Health Reform." *Health Affairs* 13: 142–56.

Cleary, P., and S. Edgman-Levitan. 1997. "Health Care Quality: Incorporating Consumer Perspectives." *JAMA* 277:1608.

Dallek, G., and N. Hasenberg. 1997. *Update of HCFA Regulations on Physician Incentive Plans.* Washington, D.C.: Families USA Foundation.

Drake, D. 1997. "Managed Care: A Product of Market Dynamics." *JAMA* 277:560–63.

Enthoven, A. 1993. "The History and Principles of Managed Competition." *Health Affairs* 12 (supp):24–48.

Enthoven, A., and S. Singer. 1997. "Markets and Collective Action in Regulating Managed Care." *Health Affairs* 16: 26–32.

Epstein, A. 1998. "Rolling the Runway: The Challenges Ahead for Quality Report Cards." *JAMA* 279:1691–96.

Families USA. 1998. "Hit and Miss: State Managed Care Laws." Washington, D.C.: Families USA Foundation (http://epn.org/families.html).

Farrell, M. 1997. "ERISA Preemption and Regulation of Managed Health Care: The Case for Managed Federalism." *American Journal of Law and Medicine* 23:251–89.

Furrow, B., et al. 1997. *Health Law Cases Materials and Problems.* 3d ed. St. Paul, Minn.: West Group.

Gabel, J. 1997. "10 Ways HMOs Have Changed During the 1990s." *Health Affairs* 16: 134–45.

Gold, M., et al. 1995. "A National Survey of Arrangements Managed-Care Plans Make with Physicians." *NEJM* 333:1670–83.

Gosfield, A. 1996. *Guide to Key Legal Issues in Managed Care Quality.* New York: Faulkner and Gray.

———. 1997. "Who Is Holding Whom Accountable for Healthcare?" *Health Affairs* 16:26–40.

Horvath, J., and K. Snow. 1996. *Emerging Challenges in State Regulation of Prepaid Managed Care Entities.* Portland, Maine: National Academy of State Health Policy.

Iglehart, J. 1997. "Health Issues, the President, and the 105th Congress." *New Eng. J. Med.* 336:671–73.

Jaklevic, M. 1996. "State Issues: A Good Year for 'Patient Protection' Laws." *Modern Healthcare* (October 28):22

Jensen, G., et al. 1997. "The Dominance of Managed Care: Insurance Trends in the 1990s." *Health Affairs* 16:125–36.

Jordan, K. 1996. "Travelers Insurance: New Support for the Argument to Restrain ERISA Preemption." *Yale Journal on Regulation* 13:255–335.

Kaufman, L., and L. Webster. 1995. "GHAA Survey Finds States Are Erratic in Oversight and Regulation of PHOs." *Health Law Reporter* 4:1063.

Kertesz, L. 1996. "Managed Care: HMOs Baling Horror Stories, Lawmakers." *Modern Healthcare* (April 8): 44–47.

Kilborn, P. 1998. "Premiums Rising for Individuals." *New York Times,* Dec. 5, p. 7A.

Kinney, E. 1996. "Procedural Protections for Patients in Capitated Health Plans." *American Journal of Law and Medicine* 22:301–30.

Kopit, W., and M. Lutes. 1993. "Legal Issues and Antitrust Considerations in the Establishment of Credentialing and Other Selection Criteria." In *The Managed Health Care Handbook,* ed. P. Kongstvedt, 2d ed. Gaithersburg, Md.: Aspen.

Lamphere, J., et al. 1997. "The Surge in Medicare Managed Care: An Update." *Health Affairs* 16:127–33.

Latham, S. 1996. "Regulation of Managed Care Incentive Payments to Physicians." *American Journal of Law and Medicine* 22:399–432.

Laudicina, S., et al. 1998. *State Legislature Health Care and Insurance Issues: 1997 Survey of Plans.* Washington, D.C.: Blue Cross Blue Shield Association.

Mariner, W. 1996. "Managed Care Regulation and the Employee Retirement Income Security Act." *New Eng. J. Med.* 335:1986–90.

Miller, R., and H. Luft. 1997. "Does Managed Care Lead to Better or Worse Quality of Care?" *Health Affairs* 16:7–23.

Miller, T. 1997. "Managed Care Regulation: In the Laboratory of the States." *JAMA* 278:1102–9.

Moran, D. 1997. "Federal Regulation of Managed Care: An Impulse in Search of a Theory?" *Health Affairs* 16:16–21.

Nather, D. 1998. "Insurance Regulation: No Mandate Seen for Patients' Bill of Rights, but Some Kind of Bill May Pass." *Health Law Reporter* 6:1777.

National Association of Insurance Commissioners (NAIC). 1996a. "Managed Care Plan Network Adequacy Model Act; Health Care Grievance Procedure Model Act; Utilization Review Model Act" (adopted by NAIC Sept. 30, 1996). Available online at www.naic.org/1papers/models.

———. 1996b. "Draft White Paper on Risk-Bearing Entities" (Sept. 24, 1996). Reprinted in *Health Law Reporter* 6:73.

Overbey, A., and M. Hall. 1996. "Insurance Regulation of Providers That Bear Risk." *American Journal of Law and Medicine* 22:361–87.

Page, L. 1996. "State Legislatures Spent Busy Year Trying to Manage Managed Care." *American Medical News,* Sept. 9, p. 6.

———. 1998. "Maryland Board: Hold HMO Medical Directors Accountable." *American Medical News,* Feb. 9, p. 1.

Parmet, W. 1993. "Regulation and Federalism: Legal Impediments to State Health Care Reform." *American Journal of Law and Medicine* 19:121–43.

Pear, R. 1998. "Health Panel at Standstill on Enforcing Bill of Rights." *New York Times,* Mar. 9, p. 12A.

Physician Payment Review Commission. 1995. "Annual Report." Washington, D.C.: U.S. Government Printing Office.

Polzer, K., and P. Butler. 1997. "Employee Health Plan Protections Under ERISA: How Well Are Consumers Protected Under Managed Care and 'Self-Insured' Employer Insurance Plans?" *Health Affairs* 16:93–102.

Riley, T. 1997. "Perspective: The Role of the States in Accountability for Quality." *Health Affairs* 16:41–43.

Robinson, J. 1996. "The Dynamics and Limits of Corporate Growth in Health Care." *Health Affairs* 15:155–67.

———. 1998. "Use and Abuse of the Medical Loss Ratio to Measure Health Plan Performance." *Health Affairs* 16:176–87.

Rodwin, M. 1996. "Consumer Protection and Managed Care Issues, Reform Proposals, and Trade-Offs." *Hous. L. Rev.* 32:1321–81.

Schneider, E., and A. Epstein. 1998. "Patient Use of Public Performance Reports: A Survey of Patients Undergoing Cardiac Surgery." *JAMA* 279:1638–42.

Shortell, S. 1994. "The New World of Managed Care: Creating Organized Delivery Systems." *Health Affairs* 13:46–64.

———. 1996. *Remaking Health Care in America: Building Organized Delivery Systems.* San Francisco, Calif.: Jossey-Bass.

Studdert, D., and T. Brennan. 1997. "Deterrence in a Divided World: Emerging Problems for Malpractice Law in an Era of Managed Care." *Behavioral Sciences and the Law* 15:21–48.

Terry, K. 1998. "No Cause Terminations: Will They Go Up in Flames?" *Medical Economics* January 12, p. 130.

Turnbull, N., and N. Kane. 1998. "The Impact of Accounting and Actuarial Practice Differences on Medical Loss Ratios: An Exploratory Study of Five HMOs." Unpublished manuscript, on file with the authors.

U.S. General Accounting Office. 1997. "Managed Care: Explicit Gag Clauses Not Found in HMO Contracts, But Physicians' Concerns Remain." GAO/HEHS-97-175. Washington, D.C.: U.S. Government Printing Office.

PART 2

Views from the Trenches: Patients and Providers

CHAPTER 4

A Physician's View
from the Trenches

Clifton R. Cleaveland

A sixty-two-year-old dredging foreman with long-standing hypertension develops intense lower abdominal pain and fever. He describes the pain as the worst he has ever experienced. In the third day of his illness, he comes to my office, where examination confirms a distended, very tender abdomen with diminished bowel sounds. He is febrile and his white blood count is elevated. Abdominal X rays show multiple air-fluid levels. I admit him to the hospital with a tentative diagnosis of acute sigmoid diverticulitis and request surgical consultation. Antibiotics, intravenous fluids, and nasogastric suction constitute initial therapy. Slowly he improves. On the second day of his hospitalization, I remove the nasogastric tube and begin a clear liquid diet. The surgeon recommends continued close observation. Later that morning, an hour after the patient's first oral intake, an unidentified utilization review nurse from his managed-care organization determines that further hospitalization will not be authorized. An appeal to the company's medical director is denied.

A severely depressed female with long-standing complex hypertension responds dramatically to Prozac. Her managed-care plan delegates mental health services to a behavioral health organization. As instructed, my patient dials a toll-free number for consultation with an unidentified person with unspecified qualifications. Subsequently, the health plan notifies me that the only drug approved for use in my patient's case is amitriptyline, a previous treatment failure in my earlier care of this patient. I use samples of Prozac from pharmaceutical representatives to meet her needs.

Many clinicians feel that George Orwell is the ultimate architect of managed care in its current form. The "Big Brother" of his novel *1984* is a paradigm for the perfect utilization reviewer for a managed-care company—omniscient, unidentifiable, and beyond challenge (Orwell 1950).

The form of managed care and the extent of its penetration varied widely and wildly in the United States in 1997. While states such as California and

Minnesota had evolved sophisticated systems of managed care throughout the 1990s, other states, particularly in the Southeast, had but limited experience with this new health-care entity. As with a biopsy, where you place the needle will determine what you get. Experiences for physicians in the new health-care climate will vary from state to state and from specialty to specialty. In a single community, primary-care physicians may work under the terms of capitated contracts, while their subspecialty colleagues will be reimbursed through fee-for-service schedules. The literature dealing with physicians' experiences in managed care is rife with anecdotes that mostly reflect horror stories.

Health Care: The Way We Were

Managed care in its various forms is a response to an unsustainable pattern of medical practice. In the early 1990s medical costs had attained runaway status and we as a nation were lurching toward a meltdown in expenditures for health care. Individuals and companies alike coped with rising health insurance premiums, which increased far faster than did the cost of living. Health economists predicted the bankruptcy of the Medicare program within a few years unless additional funding or reduced services were legislated. In many states, Medicaid expenditures represented a budget buster that threatened to squeeze out other necessary societal services such as public education and welfare (Eckholm 1993; Lee, Soffel, and Luft 1992; *The Economist* 1991).

While the media extolled the latest thrilling advances in medical technology, the costs for this technology raced upward (Ginsberg 1990). Driven by insatiable public and professional demands for the latest test or treatment, costs for individual patient and outpatient diagnostic and therapeutic encounters could quickly spiral into the tens of thousands of dollars. Technological marvels stimulated entrepreneurial zeal of companies, hospitals, and physicians. The entire health-care industry was suddenly "hot," and there were few restraints on its behavior.

Despite health-care expenditures that far exceeded those of other industrialized nations, the United States lagged in virtually every measure of clinical outcome, and polls regularly showed the disaffection of most Americans for their health-care system (Blendon and Taylor 1989). Americans with health-care insurance could pick from a lavish menu of diagnostic and treatment options, but an increasing number of our citizens—35 to 40 million by various estimates—had no health insurance of any kind. Many poor Americans either worked in low-wage jobs for employers that provided no health-care benefits or cobbled together one or more part-time jobs, which were similarly bereft of any medical insurance. Among the uninsured were millions of children.

Administrative waste, needless clinical testing, abuse of health insurance by patients and providers, and outright fraud drained billions of dollars from the health-care pool. The system seemed beyond control. Indeed, our entire health-care system resembled a brittle diabetic patient with an uncontrollable and insatiable appetite that would assure a calamitous outcome; the only question was *when.*

Health Reform Proposals from the American College of Physicians

In 1990, after years of study, analysis, and discussion within the organization, the American College of Physicians (ACP), the nation's largest organization of medical specialists, published a position paper calling for an overhaul of America's health-care system. The ACP analysis highlighted these problems: inadequate access to health care, inadequate protection by health insurance, uncontrollable costs, and a burdensome bureaucracy for patients and physicians. The ACP paper outlined a number of criteria for attaining a better system. Benefits should be uniform and evidence based. Both coverage and benefits should be independent of job, place of residence, or preexisting health status. Costs should be reduced by curtailing administrative waste and decreasing expenses of professional liability. The infrastructure in terms of facilities and manpower should be brought to a uniform and high level for all Americans, whether in urban, suburban, or rural locations. The system should monitor both patients and health-care providers for level of satisfaction.

After evaluating various alternative strategies, the ACP paper supported a nationally sponsored program for universal access to health insurance programs. The ACP proposal called for comprehensive rather than piecemeal reform. In summary, it stated:

> A comprehensive and coordinated program to assure access on a nationwide basis is essential. In the near term, given the urgency of the need, it should build on the strengths of existing health-care financing mechanisms. In the longer term, careful consideration of new and innovative alternatives, including some form of a nationwide financing mechanism, will be necessary. (ACP 1990)

Two years later, ACP's "Universal Insurance for American Health Care" fleshed out its earlier reform proposal, calling for mixed public and private financing for universal care (ACP 1992). All medically effective and appropriate care would be available in employer-sponsored and public-sponsored plans. The reform system would guarantee essential support for medical education and biomedical and health services research. Expenditures for medical services would be contained by a national health-care budget.

Under the ACP plan, employers could elect to enroll workers in a private insurance plan or pay a tax for enrolling them in a publicly directed health plan. The public plan would cover all retirees and Americans past the age of sixty, as well as poor and underserved populations and those individuals who, for whatever reasons, had no health insurance at all. Also, all medical expenses for an individual would fall under the public aegis when yearly medical costs exceeded $50,000. Services of public and private health plans would be indistinguishable. Since all plans would feature identical benefits, these plans would compete on the basis of quality and service.

The ACP proposal, while resulting from years of intraorganizational discussion, debate, and consensus building, nonetheless evoked animated criticism and condemnation, both within and without the organization. The proposal remains significant as a well-researched call for reform by a major physicians' organization.

In the subsequent national debate, stimulated by the Clinton proposals for health-care reform (White House Domestic Policy Council 1993), one proposal after another succumbed to intense attack from health insurance companies, advocacy groups representing small businesses and manufacturers, and political opponents of governmental regulation. The health-care issue, which seemed ready for serious debate after the congressional and presidential elections of 1992, sank beneath the media blitz led by the notorious "Harry and Louise" television spots. Although the push for a governmentally driven overhaul of our health-care system fizzled, striking changes of the status quo lay just ahead, driven by the same commercial forces that had attacked virtually all governmental proposals.

Health Care: Present Tense

My perspective on managed care derives from my experience for twenty-six years as a general internist in Chattanooga, Tennessee. This metropolitan area of 350,000 serves as a medical hub for rural and small-town populations of Georgia, Alabama, and Tennessee. Managed care in Tennessee received a jump start in January 1994, when HCFA waived Medicaid standards to permit the establishment of TennCare. This capitated program promised expanded and uniform health-care benefits for all residents of the state whose incomes fell below federal poverty standards. Blue Cross and for-profit companies established health maintenance organizations for Tennessee's poor. With TennCare as a catalyst, MCOs accelerated their organization of network HMOs, IPAs, and PPOs.

To cope with the chaotic and rapidly changing environment, the group of eight internists to which I belonged coalesced with several other primary-care practices to form a fifty-physician primary-care alliance of internists, family physicians, pediatricians, and obstetrician-gynecologists. The larger group permitted updated information systems, detailed contract analysis, and, most important, increased clout when negotiating with managed-care organizations. Subsequently, because of failing finances, our group placed itself under the administrative control of a community hospital's managed-care division. Our financial distress was due in substantial part to delays in payment for our services by health plans. My assessment of managed care is based upon this market-in-transition, supplemented by regular contact with colleagues in other states.

The hallmarks of this particular managed-care environment are chaos, consolidation, micromanagement, and unrestrained administrative misbehavior. Chaos results from multiple health-care plans, each with its own formulary, protocols, and mostly unpublicized restrictions upon patient care. Valuable time, consequently, is repeatedly drained from patient care to deal with labyrinthine mechanisms for patient referral and authorizations for services. Despite the availability of electronic systems, the typical health plan requires phone authorization for all but the simplest of studies.

The lengthy delays for telephone authorization are accompanied by streams of administrative forms. Substantial administrative and financial burdens are placed upon the office of each health-care provider. Further chaos derives from shifts of patients from one health plan to another as employers seek the cheapest possible coverage. Oftentimes patients do not know what company provides their coverage, nor do they have any idea what services and protocols are entailed.

Consolidation of multiple health-care enterprises and practices leads to a certain "group think" in which the quality of medical care sinks to the lowest common denominator. Diagnostic and therapeutic protocols become rigid; questions and criticism receive little encouragement. Competition can safeguard quality. When potential competitors are contracted into the same large entity, such as a physician-hospital organization, a vital stimulus to preserve this quality can be removed.

Micromanagement is best reflected in a recent protocol from one MCO that requires a phone consultation with an out-of-town "expert" each time therapy for *H pylori* infection is considered. Each MCO with which I deal features its own protocol and favored drug for managing diseases such as asthma, depression, hyperlipidemia, and hypertension. These changing requirements are summarized in a stream of letters and booklets, which in their sheer volume are overwhelming. The practitioner must try to adapt diagnosis and therapy to these varied protocols to avoid letters of reproof; their implied threat is that of being dropped from the list of approved physicians. Time simply does not exist to challenge each restriction of therapy with calls to the MCOs' medical directors or formulary supervisors.

Unrestrained administrative behavior reaches its zenith when a dispute arises with an MCO. In my state and in many others, based upon what I read and learn from multiple colleagues in these locations, most MCOs serve as judge, jury, and executioner when dealing with any dispute, whether this relates to patient care, a needed out-of-town referral, or an administrative conflict between physician and MCO. The MCOs seldom publicize for physicians the screens that are used to assess either inpatient or outpatient evaluation and therapy. Physicians have little recourse when an MCO falls behind in meeting its contractual financial obligations. Tennessee and many other states lack statutes to deal with MCOs. I have been frustrated repeatedly when dealing with utilization reviewers, who oftentimes are situated in another state. My state's insurance commissioner can offer little help or advice in such matters, and there does not seem to be any agency of the federal government capable of assisting in such situations in a timely manner.

The prospects for any federal help in disputes with large MCOs seem unlikely. Indeed, Secretary Donna Shalala of the Department of Health and Human Services was quoted as saying, "The decisions of HMOs are not made by governmental officials and the government has neither a role nor an interest in the decisions made by any HMO" (Pear 1997). This is especially interesting commentary as HMOs assume a larger role in the care of Medicare patients.

American College of Physicians' Survey on Managed Care

At its 1997 annual session in Philadelphia, the ACP released the results of a membership survey on managed care (ACP 1997). In a sample of 417 ACP members, 47 percent of whom were general internists and 53 percent of whom were subspecialists, 90 percent reported overall satisfaction with their medical careers. The same 90 percent also reported affiliation with at least one MCO. Typically, each physician dealt with seven different managed-care contracts. When the respondents were asked about their professional satisfaction in the managed-care arena, 10 percent reported that they were very satisfied, 47 percent were somewhat satisfied, 30 percent were not too satisfied, and 11 percent were not at all satisfied. Respondents affiliated with managed care for a greater length of time were more likely to describe themselves as satisfied. Whereas 18 percent of physicians who had worked under a managed-care contract for greater than five years stated they were very satisfied, only 6 percent of those affiliated with managed care for less than five years expressed a similar sentiment. Length of time in practice also influenced responses, with 15 percent of practitioners with twenty or more years of experience describing themselves as being very satisfied with managed care. Physicians in practice for fewer than twenty years described themselves as somewhat satisfied or not too satisfied with managed care. ACP members associated with staff and group model

HMOs were more positive in their views about the impact of managed care upon their clinical experiences.

When asked about the impact of MCOs upon their professional lives, 75 percent of respondents reported decreased clinical autonomy (versus 21 percent with no change and 2 percent with an increase). Sixty-four percent reported a decrease in the opportunity to refer and consult (versus 29 percent with no change and 4 percent with an increase). Income decreased for 50 percent of the respondents (versus 35 percent with no change and 11 percent with an increase), and 37 percent reported decreased productivity (versus 41 percent with no change and 19 percent with an increase).

When asked to list the single most important factor that caused satisfaction or dissatisfaction, the physicians who described themselves as very satisfied with their medical careers cited taking care of patients (29 percent), contact-relationship with patients (22 percent), and job satisfaction (21 percent). Physicians somewhat satisfied with their medical careers listed loss of autonomy (23 percent), taking care of patients (15 percent), contact-relationship with patients (12 percent), and high demands on time (12 percent) as dominant factors in their attitude toward their professional experiences. The 11 percent of internists who were not too or not at all satisfied reported loss of autonomy (53 percent), inadequate compensation (11 percent), and administrative paperwork burdens (11 percent) as the dominant factors underlying their attitudes toward their careers.

Within my own expanded primary-care group, the dominant concerns have been unwieldy bureaucratic burdens and the difficulties accessing adequate capital for expanding facilities and information systems without sacrificing organizational independence. My interpretation of the ACP survey is that the actual practice of clinical medicine remains a valued premium for most physicians despite the strictures and income loss imposed by MCOs.

A Need for Regulation

Many proponents of managed health care want the management to emanate from boardrooms independent of state and federal regulation. This attitude is embodied in the AAHP press release of May 12, 1997, "Putting Patients First" (1997). This trade group represents 90 percent of all MCOs. AAHP proposed four basic initiatives: physician-directed quality assessment and improvement programs, physician-developed practice guidelines, physician-guided utilization management criteria, and physician-reviewed prescription drug formularies. AAHP reaffirmed patients' rights to all information needed to "promote the right care at the right time in the right setting." Patient-physician confidentiality was reaffirmed, as was coverage for emergency medical care. While laudable in its content, "Putting Patients First" relies upon the voluntary efforts of

MCOs, and there are no penalties or enforcement mechanisms to assure compliance.

Sparked by burgeoning complaints from patients and professional groups, the 1995–96 legislative sessions at the state level saw hundreds of bills enacted to regulate the behavior of MCOs. The proposals dealt with gag clauses, point-of-service options, and liability of managed-care organizations for clinical decisions (Guglielmo 1997).

A variety of bills surfaced on the national level following passage of the Kassebaum-Kennedy Act (Kuttner 1997). Some proposals dealt with standards for insurance plans, while others addressed narrowly focused problems of a single disease entity such as hospital length of stay for patients following childbirth or a mastectomy.

As a practitioner, I shudder at the prospect of myriad, narrowly focused, health-related legislative acts and administrative decrees raining down upon us as one special interest group after another manages to sway a majority of congresspersons. The inscrutably complex Clinton Health Care Reform proposal would be dwarfed by such an outpouring of regulation. Based on my experience and multiple conversations with my partners and colleagues across the country, I propose a modest framework for federal regulation of managed care.

Regulation of Benefits

Consumers do not understand their rights and benefits in most managed-care contracts. In the same way that nutritional information can now be readily seen and understood on food goods, medical benefits must be clearly delineated in nontechnical language for the consumer. Benefits should be uniform across plans. These benefits should logically derive from expert panels of physicians and public health experts. The *U.S. Preventive Health Services Guide* (1997) stands as an excellent example of such collaborative work, as it assesses risks, benefits, and costs of a spectrum of preventive health measures. Approved physicians and facilities must be spelled out, and point-of-service options should be clearly stated together with the supplementary cost that this will entail for the consumer. The benefits should outline succinctly those therapies that will not be covered.

Regulation of Providers

"Any willing provider" regulations are complex and, though attractive from a democratic sense, become unwieldy in capitated contracts. Participation in capitated contracts involves considerable time and expense to the physician for legal and accounting consultation. Risks and rewards for participating in such contracts depend upon enforceable standards of behavior for all providers. In addition, a sufficiently large panel of patients must be available to allow the spread of actuarial risks. Thus, a provider outside of a carefully and expensively assembled network of patients and physicians would be free to scavenge lists of enrollees to pick off the healthiest and least expensive patients. A freebooting physician would also be less likely to adhere to group regulations and systems for practice efficiency and quality assurance.

National consensus and guidelines are essential in defining clinical privileges for various types of health-care providers. Professional boards of certification function well, but disagreements regarding issues of turf occur frequently between primary-care physicians and subspecialists as well as between physicians and nurse practitioners and physician's assistants. Federally appointed expert panels are the logical arbiters for defining clinical privileges.

Physicians have long needed legislative relief to establish provider-sponsored health-care networks. The Budget Conciliation Act for 1998 promises such assistance.

Regulation of Managed-Care Organizations

Patients and providers need published, clearly worded standards for the utilization and quality assurance of all modes of diagnosis and care. A bill of rights for providers and patients should be mandated, specifying due process for complaints, timely payment of MCO obligations, full disclosure of restrictions on care, and incentives and penalties for providers. MCOs must be held strictly accountable for the clinical outcomes that result from contractual protocols imposed upon provider and patient behavior.

In 1992, the Conservative Democratic Forum's task force on health-care reform proposed the Managed Competition Act of 1992 (H.R. 2015, 1992). Among the attractive features of this bill, which unfortunately received little public attention, was the encouragement through tax incentives for providers and MCOs to form accountable health plans (AHPs) that would offer a standard package of benefits, use community ratings to establish premiums, and enroll all individuals without regard to preexisting medical conditions. This proposal offered an attractive blend of market forces and regulation.

Regulation to Protect Education and Research

Both for-profit and not-for-profit MCOs have shown little appetite for supporting either medical education or research. MCOs cite the higher cost of care in teaching institutions; research is delegated increasingly to pharmaceutical firms. Public hospitals are avoided by MCOs because of their commitment to the medical care of poor and inner-city populations. An all-payer tax in the short term would assure funding for the education of physicians and other health professionals and for biomedical and health services research. Absent such support, our society could be likened to the tribe that devoured its seed corn.

Federal versus State Regulation

Regulation of health care in all of its complex dimensions is best handled on the federal level. The Medicare program serves as a useful model in this regard. That program would have been hopelessly fragmented had each state been accorded a block grant to care for the elderly and disabled within its borders. The wide variations in quality, services, and financing in the Medicaid programs of the various states reflect the disadvantage of decentralizing the regulation of health care. In my experience, southeastern states in particular lack the experience and skilled governmental personnel to supervise something as complex as health care.

The Daunting Issue of Quality

MCOs have succeeded in varying degrees in reducing the costs of health-care delivery. Quality of care has received lip service in most instances. Even before the advent of managed care, physicians debated without solution how to define, measure, and enforce quality of care. Again, expert panels are the logical definers and arbiters. Quality must not be allowed to vary from one health plan to another. A uniform standard must be attained by each MCO. MCOs routinely emphasize speed and economy, but quality must be inviolably linked to every health plan as well.

In summary, our American way of health care has spun out of control in the last decade. An unruly and unregulated profit-driven system of managed care has for the moment curtailed cost, but regulation and accountability must be addressed at the highest levels of government if the new kid on the health-care block is to be prevented from evolving into an overpowering bully. Following the enactment of a basic framework of regulated managed care, society must work at the even tougher issues of a national consensus on alternative health care, access to experimental therapies, and right-to-die and right-to-live controversies. Surely a nation that has placed astronauts on the moon can devise a system of health care that will give each American affordable access to compassionately delivered, scientifically based care.

REFERENCES

American Association of Health Plans (AAHP). 1997. "Putting Patients First." Press release, May 12.
American College of Physicians (ACP). 1990. "Access to Health Care." *Annals of Internal Medicine* 112:641–61.
———. 1992. "Universal Insurance for American Health Care." *Annals of Internal Medicine* 117:511–19.

————. 1997. Unpublished survey presented at American College of Physicians Annual Session in Philadelphia.

Blendon, R. J., and H. Taylor. 1989. "Views on Health Care: Public Opinion in Three Nations." *Health Affairs* 8(1): 149–57.

Eckholm, E., ed. 1993. *Solving America's Health-Care Crisis.* New York: Times Books.

Ginsberg, E. 1990. "High-Tech Medicine and Rising Health Care Costs." *JAMA* 263:1820–22.

Guglielmo, W. J. 1997. "Roping Down Managed Care." *Med. Economics* 74:106–20.

H.R. 2015, 1992.

H.R. 5936, 1992.

Kuttner, R. 1997. "The Kassebaum-Kennedy Bill—The Limits of Incrementalism." *New England Journal of Medicine* 337:64–67.

Lee, P. R., D. Soffel, and H. S. Luft. 1992. "Costs and Coverage—Pressures toward Health Care Reform." *West. J. Med.* 157:576–83.

Orwell, George. 1950. *1984.* New York: Signet Classics.

Pear, Robert. 1997. "HMOs Limiting Medicare Appeals." *New York Times,* Mar. 18.

Survey, 1991. "Surgery Needed; Last of the Big Spenders." *The Economist,* July 6, 1991, pp. 9–11.

U.S. Preventive Health Services Guide. 1997. Washington, D.C.: U.S. Government Printing Office.

White House Domestic Policy Council. 1993. *Health Security: The President's Report to the American People.* New York: Simon and Schuster.

CHAPTER 5

A Consumer Advocate's View from the Trenches

Cathy L. Hurwit

Consumer concerns about health-care quality certainly predate the rise of managed care. In the days when indemnity insurance was dominant, consumers faced quality threats from overutilization, particularly the provision of unnecessary and inappropriate services. The lack of care coordination created confusion, allowed for duplication, and meant that in many instances no one was responsible for overseeing the overall health of patients. The lack of clinically based practice guidelines meant that medical practices were not always up-to-date but were difficult to influence. Finally, many consumers had enormous difficulties getting indemnity insurers to pay for the cost of care and faced large out-of-pocket costs for care that they did receive.

Today, there are still serious concerns about consumer protections and quality; but, with the rise and current dominance of managed care, those concerns are quite different. The growth of managed care, both in public programs such as Medicare and Medicaid and in the private market, has been dramatic. Over three-quarters of privately insured workers and their families are enrolled in some form of managed care. The number of Medicaid managed-care enrollees more than doubled between 1993 and 1996, to nearly 40 percent of all beneficiaries. Roughly 100,000 Medicare beneficiaries each month are enrolling in HMOs.

In theory, managed care is supposed to correct the problems in the indemnity market, so it is not the rise in managed-care enrollment itself that creates concern. In theory, managed care is supposed to be based on improving patient care through integrated delivery systems: avoiding the problems of overutilization, establishing consumer-responsive care coordination, and improving medical practices. The problem is that, in too many instances, the theory does not reflect the reality of managed care. As a result, consumers are facing the mirror image of the problems found in the indemnity market. The failure of managed care to live up to its promise is the result of several factors.

Managed Care: Controlling Premium Costs versus Improving Health

The first factor is that managed care is too often seen primarily as a way of controlling premium costs instead of as a way of improving health outcomes. If the goal of limiting premium cost increases is paramount, then the scale is too often tilted against the consumer interest. As Victor Fuchs (1997) has written: "Managed care was a response to pressure from private and public purchasers to slow the expenditures explosion. . . . The pursuit of quality has played a minimal role." The result has been a diminution of quality as well as of affordability and access, leading to charges of health-care rationing. Because the focus has been on reducing premiums, deductibles and cost-sharing requirements have increased instead, resulting in higher consumer out-of-pocket costs. In a recent *Health Affairs* article, researcher Jon Gabel (1997), for example, reports a tripling of physician visit co-payments in HMOs over the past ten years and an increase in hospital co-payments from $4.50 to $24.90 a day. This increased cost shifting to consumers might keep premium rate increases down, but it also creates financial barriers for consumers and, as Gabel points out, a reduction in primary care.

Managed Care: Profits versus Improving the Health-Care Delivery System

The second factor is that managed care is too often seen as a way to reap enormous profits rather than as a mechanism for improving the health-care delivery system. The rise of for-profit managed care has been extraordinary. In 1981, not-for-profit HMOs represented 76 percent of market share; by 1994 they accounted for only 31 percent. There are ample indications that the rise of for-profit managed-care plans has negative consequences for consumers. Surveys by the California Medical Association have found that for-profit HMOs are likely to spend fewer premium dollars on direct patient care. For-profit HMOs are less likely to appear on the lists of highest quality plans. For instance, the highest rated HMOs listed by *Consumer Reports* ("How Does Your HMO Stack Up?" 1999) were all not-for-profit plans. To the extent that for-profit managed-care plans are less likely to be group or staff model HMOs, the ability to improve quality by influencing the practices of participating providers practicing in loose network arrangements is also diminished.

Accountability Issues

Finally, there are the overriding questions of whether managed-care plans are accountable to consumers, purchasers, or investors and whether physicians and health-care professionals are accountable to their patients or to hospital and plan administrators seeking to improve their bottom line. With the recent spate of mergers and acquisitions, large national managed-care plans have emerged; over half of all HMO enrollment is in eleven plans, for example. This trend reduces accountability not just to individuals but to entire communities, often divorcing the locus of decision making from local consumers and providers to corporations located sometimes states away. In response, consumer advocates are pursuing a strategy of mandatory community benefits, requiring that managed-care entities develop plans to improve the strength of the local delivery system, contribute to research efforts, consider the health of the entire community, and even participate in caring for the uninsured.

As a result of these factors, among others, many managed-care consumers are facing serious problems. Some of these are similar to the problems faced in the indemnity market, such as claims denials, marketing abuses, and medical malpractice committed by individual providers and hospitals. Other problems are either exacerbated or created by managed care. Those include the following:

Consumer choice. In the vast majority of cases, the consumers of health care are not the actual purchasers of health care. In the indemnity market, businesses can select a plan, but consumers can still select their hospitals, physicians, and other providers. In the managed-care market, employers select not just the plan but often, through that selection, the providers available to consumers. This not only restricts choice but, as employees change jobs and employers switch plans, also disrupts continuity of care. Both problems are particularly serious for persons with disabilities and chronic health problems. Both are exacerbated when employers offer only one plan, as do 84 percent of firms with less than five hundred employees and one-third of large employers.

Discrimination. Indemnity and managed-care plans share a common financial incentive to avoid high-cost patients. But, under managed care, providers also face those incentives through means such as financial compensation payments, including individual capitation, as well as economic profiling. Accepting high-cost patients, therefore, can result in reduced income or even loss of employment.

Denials of treatment. In the indemnity market, consumers often have difficulty obtaining payment for services that have been provided. In managed care, consumers face difficulties in obtaining the services themselves. In some cases, this may eliminate the provision of inappropriate care, but in many other instances it prevents consumers from obtaining needed treatment.

Erosion of patient-provider trust. The rise of managed care has created serious tensions between patients and providers. Instead of seeing their physicians as their advocates, patients now have to wonder whether care is being withheld because doctors may earn more by doing less. On the other hand, physicians may see high-risk patients as threats to their economic well-being. As the *Journal of the American Medical Association* (1995) editorialized: "by creating conflicting loyalties for the physician, some of the techniques of managed care can undermine the physician's fundamental obligation to serve as patient advocate."

Consumer confidence in the health-care system is further shaken by surveys of health-care professionals and patients. Among them are the following:

- According to "The Commonwealth Fund Survey of Physician Experiences with Managed Care" (1997), 60 percent of physicians in managed care reported "very or somewhat serious problems with external reviews and with limitations on their clinical decisions"; 18 percent were dissatisfied with the ability to make the right decisions for their patients; and 29 percent were dissatisfied with the amount of time available to spend with patients. Over 20 percent of physicians with more than half of their patients in managed care reported direct incentives not to refer. Only one in four were very satisfied with the practice of medicine. Dissatisfaction increased with the percentage of patients in managed care (except for physicians in group or staff HMOs, where satisfaction was generally higher except for the amount of time allowed to spend with patients).
- In New Jersey, 95 percent of nurses surveyed reported that quality of care has fallen, with 94 percent citing inadequate staffing, 71 percent delays in providing basic care, and 68 percent problems with inexperienced staff. In a national survey (Federation of Nurses and Health Professionals 1997), 37 percent of nurses said that they "would not send a family member to the hospital where they were employed."
- Families in poor health are more likely to rate managed care lower in terms of accessibility to specialists, while 20 percent of Medicare managed-care enrollees gave their plans fair or poor ratings (compared to 13 percent of fee-for-service enrollees) and 26 percent rated their physicians as fair or poor (compared to 9 percent of fee-for-service enrollees) (Commonwealth Fund 1996).
- A four-year study of patients in fee-for-service and managed-care plans found that, while average patients received similar care, senior citizens and chronically ill low-income persons were substantially better off in fee-for-service settings (Ware et al. 1996).

In short, consumers are concerned that they are being seen more as commodities than as individuals, that physicians and other health-care professionals are being restricted in what care they provide, and that the industry is putting profits—not patients—first.

The Consumer Response

Just as consumers have sought to mitigate and eliminate the problems in the indemnity market, consumers have responded to the ongoing and new issues created by the rise of managed care. Across the country, efforts to enact Managed-Care Consumers' Bills of Rights are under way. Many state legislatures or regulatory authorities have adopted portions of the Bill of Rights outlined in the following list, at the urging of consumer advocates and those within the medical community.

It is important to understand the rationale for using the Bill of Rights as a model. For consumers, the phrase has a range of very important meanings. First, a Bill of Rights is designed to protect each and every individual, not just the majority of the population. In a health-care world in which a small percentage of individuals represents a high percentage of use, this precept is critical. Second, a Bill of Rights creates protections that apply equally, regardless of circumstances such as income, health status, age, sex, race, or geographic location. Finally, a Bill of Rights provides protections that can be enforced legally, by both publicly accountable entities and individuals through legally established rights of private enforcement. Rights are created and established; protections are not dependent on the willingness of a private entity to provide them.

The principles embodied in the Bill of Rights are based on the belief that comprehensive, systemic reform is preferable to piecemeal efforts, particularly the "body-part by body-part" approaches that, while providing limited relief in very specific situations, would require years and much micromanagement to implement. For example, rather than actually setting utilization guidelines, as has been done in state and federal "anti-drive-through delivery" legislation, the Bill of Rights seeks to address the underpinnings of utilization review itself, requiring that reviewers be qualified, that protocols be based on the best available clinical evidence, and that payments not encourage adverse determinations.

In addition, the following concepts are necessary in order to ensure that the Bill of Rights meets its overall objectives:

- The Bill of Rights must be drafted in light of the needs of persons with disabilities or chronic health-care problems as well as senior citizens and low-income persons. It is not sufficient to have a health-care system that works for the currently healthy; it must work for those most vulnerable to health-care abuses because they have the highest health-care needs.
- In order to be rights, rights must be enforceable. Voluntary enforcement, disclosure of whether rights are being met, or other "market-based" proposals are not sufficient. Consumers need to know that they will enjoy a basic level of consumer and quality protections. This is particularly important because so many consumers have no ability to select their own plans

and because those who do select for them are not prohibited from enrolling them in substandard plans.

- There are no rights unless there are also remedies. Unless managed-care plans and other health-care entities can be held accountable for their actions, the ability to ensure that rights are actually provided will be greatly diminished. Moreover, unless managed-care plans are held accountable when they (or entities with which they contract) make treatment decisions, the incentive to put quality ahead of cost cutting is diminished. It is essential that consumers, physicians, nurses, and other health-care professionals and workers have the right to act on their own behalf, be given full due process rights, and have the ability to enforce accountability.

- Rights should apply to all consumers, whether they are in private or public coverage, whether they are covered by ERISA plans or commercial insurance, and whether plans are owned by providers or by Masters in Business Administration (MBAs). Regardless of the payment source, all health-care consumers deserve basic levels of protection.

- Rights should apply to all plans, wherever applicable. While the rights outlined here apply to managed-care plans, many of the consumer and quality protections could and should be provided for enrollees in fee-for-service plans as well. Moreover, rights should not be reduced because managed-care plans are operated by providers, as has been proposed by some. Because the incentives in managed-care plans are the same regardless of whether ownership is held by a hospital chain like Columbia/HCA, a company like United Health Care, or a smaller entity, the consumer and quality protections must be the same.

- The consumer protection and quality rights established must address all parts of the health-care system. It is not sufficient to set standards for managed-care plans to meet; those entities that actually provide health-care services must also be required to meet them as well. Hospitals, nursing homes, laboratories, and other facilities in particular must be held to staffing quality and adequacy standards as well as be required to protect the rights of patients, providers, and health-care workers.

- The rights established must correct the problems and emphasize the potential benefits of managed care, not return to the problems of the indemnity system. Consumers would not benefit from a return to a fee-for-service situation in which providers receive incentives to overtreat and there are no mechanisms in place to improve care coordination and appropriateness. Any willing provider laws, for instance, are one response to managed-care plans that provide access to less than adequate numbers and types of providers. An alternative approach, and one that might serve consumers better, would be to condition managed-care licensure upon a demonstration of provider network adequacy, based on the characteristics of the likely enrollee base.

The proposals promoted by consumer advocates across the country typically incorporate these concepts, although they vary in their specifics. In general, however, they include the following key rights.

The right to have timely access to appropriate care. Consumers need timely access within a reasonable travel time to a full range of culturally appropriate providers—primary care providers and specialists—within networks of the managed-care plans. Consumers need access to specialists by referral and, for people with special needs, as their care coordinator. Consumers need access to, and communities need protection for, essential community providers and specialized care centers. The assurance of appropriate access requires meeting individuals' needs but also guaranteeing the presence of a strong and responsive delivery network within the community.

The right to an affordable choice of qualified health-care professionals. In order to operate within a service area, managed-care plans must demonstrate that they have an adequate number, interdisciplinary mix, and geographic distribution of providers. Consumers should be able to choose from among health providers within a plan, including appropriate primary care providers as gatekeepers and specialists for referrals. Persons with ongoing health-care needs should have the right to use a specialist as a gatekeeper or primary provider or to obtain standing referrals. Women deserve direct access to obstetrical-gynecological care. Consumers should be able to choose health providers outside of a plan if appropriate. Consumers should have the right to choose among qualified health-care plans, with multiple options and ideally with individuals, rather than employers or public entities, allowed to make selections.

The right to comprehensive health-care benefits that meet consumers' health-care needs. Consumers should be assured that utilization review decisions are based on medical appropriateness and made by qualified professionals. Financial incentives that encourage denials, reductions, or termination of appropriate care must not be imposed either on health-care professionals or utilization reviewers. Ultimately, utilization review should be based on practice profiles, not case-by-case decisions, so that providers have some latitude to deal with their patients' unique needs, while the ability to influence the behavior of providers who routinely make inappropriate treatment decisions is retained. Consumers should have access to emergency services and, based on a prudent layperson's definition of an emergency, should be able to obtain services from the most accessible providers, regardless of whether that provider is in the plan and without need for prior approval. Consumers should have access to appropriate experimental treatments.

The right to receive health care that is affordable and free of financial barriers that impede access to it. To avoid financial barriers for all consumers, there should be limits on deductibles and other out-of-pocket costs for both in-network and out-of-network services, without discrimination among services (including the need for parity between physical and mental health services). Cost sharing should be prohibited for persons with incomes below the poverty level. Consumers' total out-of-pocket costs should be limited to affordable levels, and annual or lifetime caps must be reasonable and not impose significant financial burdens on those who experience serious illness or injury. Out-of-network costs should be the same as in-network costs for emergency care, when in-network care is not promptly available, or for new enrollees under a specialist's care for a serious health condition. Plans should be required to spend a minimum percentage of premium dollars on direct health services.

The right to high-quality care. Consumers should be guaranteed that their plans meet quality assurance standards, which include monitoring of performance and outcomes-based standards, uniform data collection and reporting, appeals and grievance procedures, the requirement of corrective actions, and participation by plan enrollees and providers. Each plan should be surveyed by an independent entity to audit quality and to determine the causes for disenrollment. The persons or entities with which the plan contracts—including hospitals, laboratories, and individual health-care professionals—must also be required to meet quality standards. Private accreditation must not substitute for public review, although duplication of effort should be avoided wherever possible.

The right to challenge decisions a plan makes about any practices or services that impact access to and quality of health care. Consumers should be guaranteed the right to challenge a broad range of decisions that can affect their health and safety, through both internal and external grievance procedures and through legal remedies. Managed-care consumers must be able to hold plans accountable and recover damages for any injuries suffered as a result of inappropriate decisions to deny, terminate, or reduce services. The courts should also have the ability to impose punitive damages where warranted. Under the external process, decisions should be based on review by a neutral third party. Consumers shall be given written notification of adverse decisions and the right to adequate representation. A patients' advocacy office should be created to assist consumers in utilizing their rights. Health-care professionals should also be given due process rights as well as whistle-blower protections.

The right to accurate, current, and understandable information about a managed-care plan. At a minimum, consumers must be provided with information on plan structure, benefits, cost-sharing requirements, numbers, and types of providers, appeals procedures, decision-making procedures, waiting times, quality measures, reasons for disenrollment, and consumer rights and responsibilities. Information should be provided in a uniform form to ensure accuracy, comprehensibility, and comparability across plans. Door-to-door marketing, financial awards for enrollment, and misleading practices should be outlawed, while independent marketing and enrollment entities should be encouraged. State and federal regulatory entities should have access to all data, in a standardized format, necessary to ensure compliance and improved quality.

The right to have medical information remain confidential and not to be discriminated against by their managed-care plan. Plans should be prohibited from discriminating against enrollees or against providers based on their or their patients' characteristics. Confidentiality of medical records should be preserved through the use of unique identifiers that allow critical data to be collected and analyzed but that cannot be used to identify specific patients. Information on enrollees should not be released to employers or others without authorization.

The right to be represented in decision making and in the organization and regulation of managed care. Enrollees should be able to participate in plan decision making through representation on the plan's governing structure or a consumer advisory board. Consumer representatives should be supported with staff and financial resources. A consumer oversight board should be established to review and monitor overall managed-care regulation and a consumer advocate should be appointed to represent consumers before regulatory bodies and in disputes with managed-care entities. A stable funding source for consumer advocacy must be created.

The right to vigorous enforcement of the Managed-Care Consumers' Bill of Rights. Consumers should be assured that quality standards are enforced, through certification of the plan as a condition of operation, external review, and individual enforcement rights. Enrollees should be provided with third-party beneficiary status and private rights of action in order to provide them with the tools to enforce those standards.

Some of the rights outlined here may appear to be similar to those included in voluntary programs such as the American Association of Health Plans' "Putting Patients First" initiative. But there are several critical differences between the Bill of Rights and voluntary approaches.

First, the Bill of Rights provides enforceable standards that are subject to neither the willingness of managed-care plans to adopt nor the ability of a "sharp shopper" to search out. These are minimum standards that all plans would be required to meet and that would be applicable to all managed-care enrollees.

Second, the Bill of Rights does not set standards that are implemented and enforced solely by the managed-care plans. While managed-care plans themselves are required to implement consumer protection and quality measures, the determination of whether plans are meeting standards is ultimately left to a publicly accountable entity through certification requirements and external quality review.

Reliance on voluntarism and the market simply will not work. The specialized nature of health care means that reliance on an "informed consumer" will often work against patients, even if consumers were given the right to choose their own insurers (which, it must be pointed out, still may limit their choice of providers to the plan's network). Given the myriad of medical services, the specific concerns of each individual, and the number of providers within each plan, there is no feasible way to provide every potential enrollee with all the information needed to ensure selection of the highest quality, appropriate plan. Assume, for instance, that quality could be adequately measured and that a consumer could choose between Plan A and Plan B. Plan A scores higher on mental health services but is below average on maternity care. Plan B is the reverse. If the consumer needs both services, how is she to choose? Instead, just as restaurants must be certified by the state health departments, managed-care plans should be certified so that minimum health and safety standards are guaranteed.

Third, consumers and the health-care professionals who care for them are given due process rights in order to ensure both that individuals are protected and that individuals can influence the practices of managed-care plans. These legal remedies are missing from voluntary approaches and in today's market.

Fourth, consumers and health-care professionals are guaranteed a participatory role in the health-care system, including representation and inclusion in adopting clinical protocols. Under voluntarism and the market, plans remain in control. Under the Bill of Rights, control and accountability are shared.

Conclusion

The Bill of Rights approach is designed to assure that managed-care participants receive high-quality, accessible health care. It does not represent a full-scale solution to the nation's health-care problems. Those problems include an uninsured population that makes the United States unique among industrialized countries; the world's most expensive system that increasingly shifts costs to individuals and families; and a lack of access to all needed benefits (including Medicare, which fails to provide prescription drug or long-term care services so vital to senior citizens and persons with disabilities). These problems, if they are to be solved, require comprehensive and systemic action. Ultimately, if we are to be successful, the United States will have to decouple access to health care from employment status or income. The solution lies in building upon the Medicare social insurance model to provide an improved Medicare (both through expanded benefits and reduced individual out-of-pocket costs) for all Americans.

REFERENCES

Clancy, C., and Brody, H. 1995. "Managed Care: Jekyll or Hyde?" *JAMA* 273:338–39 (January 25) (editorial).

Commonwealth Fund. 1996. *Annual Report*. New York. Commonwealth Fund.

Commonwealth Fund. 1997. Survey of Physician Experienced with Managed Care. New York. Commonwealth Fund.

Federation of Nurses and Health Professionals, American Federation of Teachers. 1997. "The Incredible Shrinking Health Care Staff: Protecting Quality Standards in a Bottom-Line Environment." Washington, D.C.: American Federation of Teachers, AFL-CIO.

Fuchs, Victor. 1997. "Managed Care and Merger Mania." *JAMA* 277:920–21 (March 19).

Gabel, Jon. 1997. "Ten Ways HMOs Have Changed During the 1990s." *Health Affairs* 16: 134–45.

"How does your HMO stack up?" *Consumer Reports,* August 1999.

Ware, J., et al. 1996. "Differences in 4-Year Health Outcomes for Elderly and Chronically Ill Patients Treated in HMO and Fee-for-Service Systems." *JAMA* 276:1039–47 (October 2).

CHAPTER 6

Oversight of Managed Care: An Academic Health Center Perspective

John E. Billi and Jeanne M. Kin

The nation's academic health centers—medical schools and their affiliated teaching hospitals—are an essential societal resource. Academic health centers

- educate future physicians, nurses, allied health professionals, and biomedical scientists;
- create new knowledge through basic biomedical research and clinical research;
- evaluate new medical treatments and technology and disseminate them to the community; and
- provide a full spectrum of patient care services, including specialized services and cutting-edge tertiary and quaternary care.

Academic centers' clinical programs have traditionally been organized around the provision of high-tech, specialty, and inpatient tertiary services (Sinaiko 1996). Special services more likely to be found in a teaching hospital include advanced cardiac care, care of AIDS patients, cancer research and treatment, trauma care, transplants, geriatrics, and specialized intensive care units (e.g., burn, neonatal, pediatric) (AAMC 1998a). The specialized services, latest technology, clinical research trials, and expertise available at academic health centers attract a sicker, more complex subset of patients than those cared for at nonteaching hospitals, including patients with rare conditions and those transferred from other hospitals (Moy et al. 1996a; Blumenthal, Campbell, and Weissman 1997).

The academic health center's social mission also embraces care to the medically underserved. Faculty practice plans and teaching hospitals, especially publicly owned facilities, are critical providers of health-care services to uninsured and indigent populations in urban centers and in rural areas (Moy 1998b). Major teaching hospitals represent only 6 percent of the nation's hospitals but provide nearly 50 percent of all charity care (AAMC 1998a). Charity care charges per physician member of a faculty practice plan averaged about $32,000 in 1997 and continue to rise (Valente and Serrin 1998). Teaching hospitals also provide significantly more care to Medicaid beneficiaries than do nonteaching institutions (Moy 1998b). Reimbursement for Medicaid services is frequently at rates lower than other payers (Physician Payment Review Commission 1994). Academic health centers' costs of providing uncompensated care (charity care plus bad debt) are increasing, and, on average, less than one-quarter of the costs of providing uncompensated care is offset by government appropriations (AAMC 1997).

Academic health centers, with their multiple, interrelated missions, roles, affiliations, and constituencies, are organizationally and financially complex institutions. An academic health center can simultaneously function as school, research institute, integrated clinical delivery system or integrated delivery network, hospital, outpatient practice network, physician group practice, physician organization or independent practice association, outpatient diagnostic facility, and, in recent years, managed-care organization. The research, teaching, and clinical care missions of academic health centers are interwoven in a web of financial cross-support, with patient care the only activity that generates a positive margin (Moy et al. 1996b; Gold 1996). The structure and culture of the academic health center are a hybrid of academic and corporate management styles and values (Blake 1996).

Academic health centers face an uncertain future because their multiple roles make them "non-competitive in a price-sensitive environment" (Foreman 1994). Eighty-five percent of the insured workforce is now in some type of managed-care plan (AAMC 1998f), and the number of Medicaid and Medicare beneficiaries who voluntarily enroll in or are required to join managed-care plans is growing (Iglehart 1999a, 1999b). As managed care has emerged as the dominant model of health care across the country, patient volumes and clinical financial margins at academic health centers have been endangered or reduced (Kassirer 1994). Many academic health centers do not have the base of primary care providers essential to success in managed care. The teaching hospital component of the academic center has been particularly threatened as the delivery of health care has progressively shifted to more cost-effective ambulatory settings (Blake 1996).

At the same time as clinical income is declining, other traditional sources of funding for medical schools' and teaching hospitals' mission-related costs are under pressure. Special payments from the Medicare program and from state Medicaid programs have historically helped balance academic health centers' costs associated with medical education, research, and uncompensated care (AAMC 1998b). These payments are now the target of reductions intended to close funding gaps in state and federal budgets. In July 1996, the Health Care Financing Administration implemented new billing guidelines that restricted the ability of teaching physicians to bill Medicare for their professional services while educating and supervising trainees (Sinaiko 1996). The rate of increase for funding of research through the National Institutes of Health (NIH), the major source of support for biomedical and behavioral research at medical schools and teaching hospitals, has declined in recent years (AAMC 1999d). (The Association of American Medical Colleges [AAMC] and other advocacy groups are advocating vigorously for a doubling in the NIH budget by 2003). One need look no further than the media headlines ("Teaching Hospitals in Trouble" 1999) to appreciate that teaching hospitals in major cities around the country—Boston, New York, Chicago, Washington, D.C., San Francisco, Providence, Detroit, Dayton, Philadelphia—are in financial distress (AAMC 1998e).

The public, when asked its opinion, does appear to value the contributions academic health centers make to society (AAMC 1996a). Advances in medical research and well-trained health-care practitioners are particularly highly regarded. It is perplexing, then, that no public policy mantle protects academic health centers' missions from the forces of market competition (Blumenthal, Campbell, and Weissman 1997). The public and its representatives may not understand the role teaching hospitals and medical schools play in serving the health-care needs of the nation, or they may not appreciate that these extraordinary institutions are threatened.

This chapter will explore how competitive pressures are affecting the missions of academic health centers; describe how academic health centers are responding to the challenges of the managed-care marketplace; provide the academic health center's perspective on the oversight and regulation of managed care; and conclude with an approach to preserving the vital public missions of academic health centers.

Academic Health Centers in the Managed-Care Era

A recent article in *Academic Medicine* on the meeting of managed care and academic medicine was aptly subtitled "A High Impact Collision" (Carey and Engelhard 1996). As cost-containment pressures in the health-care market have driven down profit margins on clinical care, a consequence (whether intended or unintended) has been the withdrawal of an important source of indirect subsidies for public health-care goods and services produced by academic health centers (Blumenthal and Meyer 1996). The Commonwealth Fund Task Force on Academic Health Centers estimated that the social missions of research, education, and specialized care added more than $18 billion to the price tag for patient care in 1997 (Commonwealth 1998). Academic health centers are finding it increasingly difficult to support their public and academic missions with income from clinical activities (Biles and Simon 1996), which they were able to do in the less constrained era of fee-for-service reimbursement.

Most managed-care organizations have limited or no commitment to supporting the education, research, and charity care missions of academic health centers (AAMC 1999d). Managed-care organizations and other cost-sensitive purchasers base their purchasing decisions on cost and quality of services for their members—with the assumption that the competitive forces of the market will result in the highest quality, most efficient providers winning market share (see chapter 8). Purchasers are not willing to pay a differential to academic health centers over other providers for their clinical services (although a small "premium," on the order of 5 to 10 percent, might be acceptable to some payers [Gold 1996], justified on the basis of patient mix, reputation of the Academic Health Center (AHC), or other factors). The implicit social contract that permitted academic centers to subsidize their social mission costs through higher charges to private insurers is no longer in force. Payers are especially unwilling to pay a differential in the absence of convincing evidence that an academic health center provides better value (defined as quality divided by price) or cares for sicker patients than do its community competitors.

Faculty at academic health centers believe they offer superior clinical quality, the rationale underlying this belief being that academic physicians are more likely to apply the latest techniques and standards of medical practice. Evidence is emerging to support this assumption (Griner 1998). But better quality outcomes of care can be difficult to document, whereas the costs of the academic center's clinical services are highly visible to those paying the bills. A 1995 study of seven academic health centers found pricing structures at teaching hospitals to be 15 to 30 percent higher for similar clinical services than the average price in the community (Blumenthal and Meyer 1996). A study undertaken by the AAMC in 1994 found that the average cost of care per admission in 1991 was about $6,000 at a teaching hospital, as compared to $4,400 at a nonteaching hospital (Dobson, Coleman, and Mechanic 1994).

These higher cost structures have put academic health centers at risk of being shut out of the managed-care networks that increasingly direct the referral of patients. In selected metropolitan areas, the share that academic centers have of the HMO market is lower than their share of the market for other privately insured patients (Reuter, Gaskin, and Hadley 1996). This diversion of patients away from academic health centers erodes revenues and reduces the number of patients available for clinical training and research (Biles and Simon 1996).

Mission versus the Market

For a variety of mission-critical reasons, academic health centers cannot afford *not* to be contenders in the managed-care arena.

Clinical Mission

Academic health centers need an adequate patient base and reimbursement to support their faculty practice plans, facilities, and delivery systems. Managed-care organizations may be interested in including teaching hospitals in their provider networks for the value of the academic center's reputation but often are willing to contract only at discounted rates and may want to contract only for the high-end specialized services not otherwise available in the community (Gold 1996). This puts the academic health center in a precarious situation: specialized, high-end services are expensive to provide and frequently lose money because reimbursement is limited compared to the cost of maintaining the service capacity (Blumenthal, Campbell, and Weissman 1997; Sinaiko 1996).

The academic health center cannot survive on revenue from tertiary care and specialized services alone. Secondary care is the bread-and-butter business that provides a measure of financial stability for teaching hospitals. In the fee-for-service era, academic centers relied on their reputations and good relations with referring physicians to deliver patients to the secondary, tertiary, and unique specialized services of their teaching hospitals. In an environment where care is increasingly directed by health plans, academic centers must have contracts with managed-care organizations to secure referrals to their secondary and tertiary services. Perhaps most important to survival, academic centers that do not have the base of primary care providers that is essential to full participation in managed care must either develop it or be part of a larger system that does have primary care capacity. Over and above financial considerations, providing the full spectrum of patient care services within an integrated academic system is highly desirable for educating health professional students.

Twin issues loom large when academic health centers pursue managed-care contracts: risk adjustment and adverse selection. Academic health centers that share financial risk or take capitation for members enrolled in managed-care plans are in serious jeopardy of adverse selection: receiving a biased, sicker subset of eligible plan members. This may be due either to the academic health center's reputation for expertise in managing the sickest patients or to a preexisting relationship with such patients when they join an HMO.

Data confirm that the average patient in a teaching hospital is significantly sicker than the average patient in other hospitals. Some of these case-mix differences between academic centers and other hospitals are captured by diagnosis-related groups (DRGs), but there is considerable variation within DRGs in both principal diagnoses and comorbidities. Within DRGs, teaching hospitals' patients tend to have principal diagnoses associated with longer lengths of stay. Within DRG and principal diagnosis pairs, teaching hospitals' patients have more severe comorbidities (Moy 1998a).

Academic health centers with their special services and disease management programs are uniquely qualified to treat the most severely ill patients, but they must be paid adequately for their patient mix. The continued availability to the public of the special services offered at academic health centers will be determined in part by the ability of academic centers to underwrite the costs of these programs. Until more sophisticated models for adjusting for case mix and severity are perfected and implemented by government and private health plans, academic health centers and the special services they offer are in jeopardy.

In a capitated environment, adverse selection is a recipe for financial disaster. If payments to academic health centers are not risk-adjusted to take into account the higher resource needs of the populations they attract, academic health centers will either go out of business or be forced to walk away from their special missions. A recent study reported that academic health centers did lose money on each managed-care contract, a deficit that was subsidized by the financial margin from care delivered to fee-for-service patients (Blumenthal 1998).

Because of their tertiary capabilities and special services, academic health centers in some markets are in the unusual position of still serving substantial numbers of fee-for-service patients. This residual fee-for-service business has buffered academic centers in some markets from experiencing the full impact of market forces and managed care. Leaders and faculty of academic centers need to understand that this is only a temporary reprieve. As managed-care penetration and more cost-sensitive patient direction increase, a strategy of preserving revenue by attracting a larger share of the dwindling fee-for-service market will not be viable over the long term.

Government programs, especially Medicare and Medicaid, have long been important payers for academic health centers. Public programs paid for 46.2 percent of health care in the United States in 1998, up from 40.5 percent in 1990 (HCFA 1998). Exposure to the Medicaid and other underserved populations is an especially important part of any teaching program. If physicians-in-training do not have opportunities to work with underserved populations, they are less likely to incorporate service to the poor into their career goals.

Medicare and, in some states, Medicaid provide explicit funding to teaching hospitals for graduate medical education (the training of residents). Medicare "direct medical education" payments, which totaled $2.2 billion in fiscal 1997, cover a share of residents' salaries, faculty salaries, and administrative expenses. Medicare "indirect medical education" payments, which totaled $4.6 billion in fiscal 1997, reflect the added costs of patient care associated with the operation of teaching programs (Iglehart 1999a). Teaching hospitals also benefit from Medicare "disproportionate share" (DSH) payments. These special payments are intended to compensate hospitals for the higher operating costs they incur in treating a large share of low-income Medicare and Medicaid patients and to preserve access to care for low-income populations by financially assisting the hospitals who serve them. DSH payments are an add-on to the DRG payments that Medicare makes to hospitals through its prospective payment system. DSH payments totaled $4.5 billion in 1997 (AAMC 1998g).

Medicare's status as the largest explicit source of financing for graduate medical education is in transition. In the Balanced Budget Act of 1997 Congress reduced Medicare "indirect medical education" payments to teaching hospitals by $5.6 billion over five years and cut "direct medical education" payments by an estimated $700 million over five years (Biles 1997; Commonwealth 1997; Iglehart 1999a). (These reductions were partially offset by returning to hospitals a portion of the premiums Medicare pays to managed-care plans). Reductions of this magnitude will have a significant adverse impact on hospitals with large teaching activity (AAMC 1999c). A recent simulation conducted by the AAMC projects that, due to the Balanced Budget Act, the median total margin for major teaching hospitals will decline to almost zero by 2002 (AAMC 1999c). The AAMC and teaching hospitals across the country are lobbying for the restoration of BBA-imposed reductions in the Medicare program, on the basis that these reductions have gone too far and threaten the long-term financial stability of U.S. teaching hospitals (AAMC 1999e). The Balanced Budget Refinement Act (BBRA) provided some relief. According to AAMC estimates, however, the typical teaching hospital will still lose over $40 million between 1998 and 2002, even with the enactment of the BBRA (AAMC 2000).

In a positive development from the academic health center's perspective, the Balanced Budget Act of 1997 does attempt for the first time to risk-adjust the premium paid to Medicare HMOs on the basis of patients' clinical characteristics (Iezzoni et al. 1998). Whether this will, in fact, result in more dollars flowing to the academic health center providers at risk for high-use members remains to be seen. Even if the HCFA does appropriately adjust Medicare premiums paid to HMOs that enroll higher resource-using members, the HMO could keep the premium differential and not pass it on to the provider at risk for delivering the care to the sicker patients.

A similar concern exists if an academic health center takes financial risk for managed Medicaid lives and the premium is not adequately adjusted. Under fee-for-service Medicaid, if reimbursement for this population were low, the academic center could pass the excess cost of caring for these patients on to their other payers through higher prices (Carli 1999). In today's managed-cared-dominated market, this cost shifting is no longer tolerated by cost-conscious payers.

Responding to Cost Reduction Pressures

Academic health centers have attempted to respond to the cost pressures of the health-care marketplace by aggressively reducing costs, reorganizing, restructuring, reengineering, and engaging in benchmarking and entrepreneurial activities in the competitive marketplace (Cyphert 1997; Griner and Blumenthal 1998). Academic health centers are employing multiple strategies to develop networks of sufficient size and geographic coverage to be attractive to managed-care plans. Medical schools and teaching hospitals are

- partnering with other providers to form integrated delivery systems;
- merging with other providers to rationalize services, eliminate redundancies, and achieve economies of scale;
- developing or acquiring a large primary care base to meet managed-care payer needs; and
- moving services out of the teaching hospital setting, which tends to be both costly and inconvenient for patients, and into more accessible, patient-friendly community settings.

As academic centers move out into the community and engage in networking, an inherent challenge for them is to maintain good relations with those referring physicians and community hospitals upon whom they have historically relied for patient referrals. Academic centers must position themselves carefully to be perceived by the community network participant as a complementary "partner in care," not a competitor. Academic centers bring reputations for quality and other, more tangible strengths to clinical networks, including expertise in evidence-based medicine, outcomes research, practice guideline development and dissemination, clinical quality improvement methods, and opportunities for participation in clinical research trials and clinical education. From a legal perspective, the structuring of networks that stop short of full integration must be approached cautiously to prevent any potential violation of antitrust laws or of Stark II regulations, which are intended to curb abuses in physician self-referral arrangements.

Another aspect of building the "academic" integrated delivery system has been the melding of clinical faculty, traditionally structured along academic departmental lines, into multidisciplinary group practices. Eliminating departmental fiefdoms and autonomous decision making at the departmental level involves a cultural upheaval for academic centers. This integration has caused tensions among different cohorts of faculty, some of whom are in traditional academic roles insulated from the forces of cost competition, while others spend most of their efforts in clinical care and clinical teaching, in the midst of the new realities. Developing a cohesive faculty group practice is a difficult but critical step in positioning academic centers to be competitive in the future.

In contrast to those academic health centers that have formed networks and grown their clinical enterprises into integrated delivery systems to be better positioned for managed care, other academic centers have divested some or all of their clinical facilities either due to financial exigencies or because they perceived the volatility and risk of the market as too high (Cerra 1997). Divestiture comes at a high price in terms of the academic center's ability to control its own destiny and discharge its academic and social missions.

Transformation of the academic health center's clinical enterprise through internal reform, restructuring, and cultural change is a necessary survival strategy. However, even if academic health centers were carrying out all of their missions at peak efficiency, informed observers do not believe that teaching hospitals would ever be able to compete with community hospitals on price alone (Blumenthal, Campbell, and Weissman 1997). The presence of interns and residents-in-training is thought to introduce inefficiencies that can never be entirely eliminated, and academic centers have the additional burdens of research, technology development and dissemination (Reuter 1997), and uncompensated care.

Education

Educating the next generation of health professionals is the academic health center's most visible social mission. To discharge this responsibility effectively, the academic health center must be immersed in new models of managing and financing care. Unless academic centers become managed-care-ready organizations, the health professionals they educate will be ill-prepared to function in the practice settings that await them on graduation.

There are specific skills and competencies a physician must master to function in managed care, including clinical prevention, risk assessment and knowledge of health care needs of populations, evidence-based medicine, quality measurement and improvement, care management, and team work (Lurie 1996; Moore 1993; AAMC 1998b). Medical schools' clinical faculty must practice in well-run, managed-care-compatible settings in order to be proficient in and able to teach these skills. Trainees practicing in settings with managed-care patients learn to function as a team with other physicians and health professionals and to manage the entire population for whom the team is responsible—not just those patients who seek care. In managed-care systems medical students and residents experience how prevention and population-based medicine can work. For example, indemnity insurers do not send their physicians a list of patients in need of mammograms; managed-care plans do.

In addition to specific managed-care competencies, medical school faculty must also ground future health professionals in ethics and professional values to prepare them for managing the ethical issues arising out of cost containment and managed care (Rodwin 1995). The public is very concerned over conflicts of interest arising from physician capitation, risk sharing, and incentives to withhold care; inculcating new physicians with high professional and ethical standards has never been more timely and important (Woolhandler and Himmelstein 1995; Relman 1992; Mechanic and Schlesinger 1996).

Given that exposure to managed care is essential to the preparation of the next generation of physicians, actions that limit academic centers' participation in managed care threaten their educational missions. Some managed-care plans are reluctant to contract with academic health centers for reasons beyond their higher costs. Plans may fear that the involvement of students and residents in patient care will interfere with efficiency and physician accountability, mainstays of the managed-care model for improving clinical care. Or there may be concern that patient satisfaction will suffer if trainees are included on the health-care team.

Market-oriented managed care can adversely affect the availability of clinical teachers and clinical teaching sites in the community. Over half of medical student education and the vast majority of residency training are carried out in clinical settings. Even the largest academic centers are not able to rely solely on their own facilities and employed faculty to deliver all clinically based education. Almost all medical schools affiliate with external providers to secure additional clinical training sites for students and residents. These affiliates range from individual volunteer faculty in private offices to entire integrated delivery systems.

As academic health centers have extended their services into the community (partly in response to managed-care pressures for primary care networks in local communities), volunteer faculty teachers may perceive the academic health center as more of a competitive threat than it was in the past. This in turn may lead to community affiliates dropping their teaching activities. Or volunteer teaching faculty may simply find that teaching impairs their productivity and may decide that involvement in teaching is a luxury they can no longer afford. Some academic centers have found it necessary to pay volunteer clinical faculty for their teaching services to compensate for the impact of teaching on productivity. Most medical schools have found it beneficial to align their clinical and educational networks to assure stability for their clinical education programs.

Research Mission

Academic health centers have been characterized as the research and development arm of the American health-care system. Biomedical research can be viewed as a continuum extending from basic science, through clinical application to patients, to studies of health and disease in populations. In academic centers, the knowledge gained in the basic science laboratory is translated into diagnostic and therapeutic applications in the clinic and at the bedside (AAMC 1998c).

Over the past fifty years federal grant funding to university investigators has established biomedical research as a core function of medical schools and has fostered a rich scientific environment for the training of physicians, biomedical researchers, and health professionals (AAMC 1999d). Most health-related research occurs in academic health centers, with over 50 percent of NIH research grants going to medical schools (Pardes 1997). In 1997 NIH awarded 16,687 grants, totaling $4.8 billion, to the 125 U.S. medical schools (AAMC 1999a). The majority of NIH grants for research training (the education of future biomedical scientists) are also awarded to academic centers (AAMC 1993).

Federal funding for biomedical research and research training is rooted in the assumption that investment in research yields major benefits for society in the form of medical advances and innovation, resulting in the improved health of Americans. It also advances the U.S. economy through the formation and growth of new technology-based industries such as biopharmaceutics or gene therapy (AAMC 1999d).

In a cost-constrained health-care system, medical advances and new technology are a mixed blessing: the benefits of medical advances and innovation are eagerly sought after by patients, but the role of technology in driving up health-care costs cannot be ignored (AAMC 1999d). Providing health-care services to a population within a fixed budget is a basic tenet of capitated managed care. But if budgets are fixed, how will consumer demand for the benefits of expensive technology be met? And who will bear the risk for making medical advances available? Rigorous technology assessment will help inform the public debate over which technological advances should be paid for out of limited resources, but it will not expand the pool of resources available to deliver care. The question of who should pay for clinical trials and experimental medical treatments is similarly controversial. Should these clinical applications of research be considered patient care, research, or both?

The long-term impact of the growth of managed care on biomedical research is uncertain. Academic leaders fear that financial pressures in the price-competitive market will result in diminution of both the clinical workforce and revenues available for research in academic centers (Cohen 1996). An AAMC survey indicated that $800 million per year, or ten cents of every faculty practice plan dollar collected, is gleaned from the clinical revenues of medical school faculty to support research (Jones and Sanderson 1996). These funds are invested in new ideas, support investigators' bridging needs between grants, and provide start-up funds for new faculty (Cohen 1996). Shrinking margins in a price-driven health care market jeopardize this internally-generated support for research. There is some evidence that academic centers in highly competitive markets are restricting their research activities. Between 1990 and 1995 research grants from the NIH to medical schools in areas with low or medium managed-care penetration rose in constant dollars; awards to schools in areas with high managed-care penetration declined (Moy et al. 1997). Many academic health centers are attempting to diversify their funding base by developing new linkages with industry and philanthropic sources of support to replace declining clinical dollars available to support research.

In this era of competitive, cost-constrained health care, academic health centers are being called upon to conduct new and different types of clinical research. The fields of outcomes and effectiveness research, decision sciences, clinical epidemiology, and quality improvement methods are coming into their own (Griner and Blumenthal 1998). Managed-care organizations are not commonly interested in supporting medical research, but they do share a keen interest with academic health centers in the field of evidence-based medicine: knowledge of what works and what doesn't in medicine. This shared interest could lead to mutually beneficial collaboration between managed-care plans and academic institutions around health services or clinical research projects relevant to the delivery of well-coordinated care.

The Academic Health Center and the Regulation of Managed Care

Academic health centers are diverse in their histories, range of functions, organizational structures and market environments. An academic health center's view of a particular means of regulating managed care will vary, depending on its role in managed care and its experience with managed-care payers in its region. For example, the academic health center that owns its own HMO will react negatively to lowering the bar for HMO licensure, while an academic health center without a managed-care plan may view this as an opportunity to diversify its payer pool. Even legislation clearly designed to benefit academic centers, such as a requirement for HMOs to contract with all teaching hospitals in their region, could be viewed negatively by an academic health center in a competitive market, if the particular center has already succeeded in negotiating exclusive contracts with one or more managed-care plan in its region.

Recognizing that different academic health centers will have divergent views on some issues, the next section provides an overview of how academic health centers might typically perceive various methods of regulating managed care.

Academic Health Center as Provider

The academic health center's fundamental relationship to managed-care organizations is as a provider. Thus the academic center's perspective on most methods of regulating managed care will mirror the views of other providers. The academic center is likely to regard favorably regulation that protects patients and providers, including minimum benefit packages, mandated coverage for preventive services, mental health parity, appeals processes for patients and providers, standards for utilization review, strict protection of patient confidentiality (provided it does not interfere with the use of data for research), and anti–gag clause provisions. Academic health centers will also favor rules that would provide coverage for care that they disproportionately provide, such as bone marrow transplant for certain malignancies or solid organ transplants.

Academic health centers and other providers of managed care have an interest in ensuring that those persons selecting a managed-care plan as their insurance choice are fully aware of the benefits, processes, and limitations of the plan prior to selection. Most academic health centers would therefore favor mandatory disclosure of information about a managed-care organization's rules and policies to enrollees, potential enrollees, and the public. Such information mandated for release can include physician financial incentives, procedures for access to specialists, how "experimental" treatments are determined, the definition of emergency services, and out-of-area benefits.

Similarly, most academic health centers would favor a requirement that managed-care organizations disclose performance data to the general public upon request, including the plan's HEDIS measures and efficiency results. Academic health centers would, certainly, have the same concerns as other providers about the accuracy of any physician or hospital profiles (quality, cost, utilization data) to be released. And academic health centers would have a particular interest in assuring that their provider identified data were appropriately risk-adjusted to reflect the sicker subset of patients attracted to such centers.

Academic Health Center as MCO

A number of academic health centers do operate a managed-care plan or are part of an integrated system that includes a health plan. These institutions will naturally share the perspective of HMOs on certain types of regulation.

An academic center with an HMO is likely to view any willing provider laws as negatively as would any other HMO owner, since such laws restrict an HMO's flexibility to contract selectively. And since one reason academic health centers may own an HMO is to ensure access to patients, any law that forces HMOs to include other providers limits this benefit to the academic center. Any willing provider laws also tend to promote competition with the academic health center's specialized services.

Academic health centers that accept insurance risk under managed care would share the concern of other capitated providers and HMOs over mandates that expand coverage by disease or diagnosis, for example, treatment of temporomandibular joint (TMJ) syndrome, without commensurate increases in premium rates. A conflict may arise between clinician faculty and financial officers within the academic health center when the benefit expansion includes highly specialized services in which faculty have special interest or research expertise (such as treatment of infertility or bone marrow transplant) without capitation adjustment or premium increase.

Several proposals for increasing accountability in managed care would hold managed-care organizations and/or their medical directors liable for the utilization and care management decisions they make. Such regulations are intended to foster more responsible decision making by the threat of tort liability or state medical board action if a bad outcome can be traced to a faulty care management decision. Under these proposals, individuals who are harmed by decisions would have recourse through private litigation or through a state process. If the academic health center owns an HMO, or might be named in such a suit as a manager of care, it would likely not favor such legislation. Since it has been shown that medical malpractice rarely identifies and holds providers accountable for poor care, it seems unlikely that subjecting managed-care decisions to the same tort process would result in more just outcomes (Localio et al. 1991)

Academic Health Center's Unique Issues

Academic centers will have a unique perspective on types of regulation that have the potential to affect them differentially.

Access
Preserving patient access to their services is a critical issue for teaching institutions. This disposes academic health centers to favor provisions such as a prudent layperson standard for coverage of emergency room services, direct access to specialists, mandatory point-of-service plan options, and "essential community provider" provisions that require managed-care organizations to contract with institutions that provide substantial amounts of care to the medically indigent.

Experimental Treatment
Coverage of experimental and investigational therapies is germane to academic centers. Academic centers would support requiring all payers to cover the full medical cost of experimental therapies associated with an NIH- or other government agency-sponsored clinical trial. The caveat that the clinical trial must be federally sponsored would guarantee peer review of the quality of the research and assure that the patient had the benefit of protections provided by an Institutional Review Board (IRB) review of the protocol. Academic health centers would also advocate for a rapid, explicit process for moving a therapy that the scientific evidence has found effective from "investigational" (not covered) to "covered benefit" status.

Nondiscrimination

Many managed-care proposals call for nondiscrimination against potential members based on prior health conditions or other characteristics. Since academic centers tend to care for the sickest populations, they would naturally favor nondiscrimination regulations such as the elimination of preexisting condition exclusions.

Discussion

This chapter has explored the daunting challenge facing academic health centers in the managed-care era: how to weather the transformation of health-care financing while preserving their valued academic and social missions. Market forces precipitated this crisis in academic medicine by placing increased pressure on the clinical margins historically used to cross-subsidize research, education, and uncompensated care.

Academic health centers must adapt to the changing system of health-care delivery and become active participants in managed care. This will require difficult internal restructuring and reform, but it is essential for both the financial survival of the academic health center and for effective discharge of its academic mission.

Even with internal reform and improved efficiency in their operations, academic health centers cannot be expected to compete in the managed-care marketplace while simultaneously subsidizing their social missions from patient care revenues. The cost-competitive nature of the health-care system has put academic health centers in the untenable position of not being able to afford to carry out their social missions. Extrication from this predicament is not, however, to be found in the regulation of managed care; governmental intervention of a different sort is required.

Preservation of the social missions of academic health centers can only be addressed in the arena of public policy. Academic health centers must demonstrate their value as a societal resource and advocate effectively for the resources needed to support the public goods and services they produce. A number of proposals have been made to level the playing field for academic health centers and teaching hospitals by supporting the higher costs of patient care associated with their social missions through all-payer pools or trust funds paid directly to the institutions themselves (Reuter 1997). An all-payer medical school fund was proposed in 1994 health-care reform legislation to help medical schools finance the incremental costs of moving clinical education to ambulatory settings and to preserve research infrastructure and capacity that were dependent on subsidies from clinical revenues (AAMC 1996b). A recent policy initiative, the *Report of the Commonwealth Foundation's Task Force on*

Academic Health Centers (Commonwealth 1998), recommends a $15 billion trust fund, separate from patient care revenue, to be financed through contributions from Medicare, Medicaid, a health insurance premium tax, and general revenues. Similar proposals have been recommended by the Prospective Payment Assessment Commission, by the Institute of Medicine, and in the 1995 Budget Reconciliation Act (which was passed by Congress but vetoed by the president). Proponents of the trust fund approach find it a reasonable compromise between protecting threatened social missions and allowing markets to function (Blumenthal and Thier 1998). This approach would allow academic health centers and other teaching hospitals to compete in the managed-care market on the basis of price, yet still pursue their vital missions. It is governmental intervention on this scale, not regulation of managed-care plans, that will ultimately be required to protect the threatened social missions of academic centers. Only the federal government is in a position to institute a formal structure whereby the many beneficiaries of academic health center programs can contribute proportionately to their support (AAMC 1996b).

With public support comes public accountability. The formulation of sound public policy will require improved collection and analysis of data to track the effects of the changing environment on the academic health centers' social missions (Blumenthal, Campbell, and Weissman 1997). Academic health centers must be prepared to demonstrate that they are carrying out their social missions in an efficient and responsible manner. They must verify that they are producing "public goods" that are relevant to the needs of society: goods such as a physician workforce comprised of an appropriate mix of primary care and specialty providers possessing the skills to function effectively and efficiently in ambulatory care and managed-care settings and new types of clinical research relevant to health-care delivery.

Oversight of managed care, although not the solution to the problems confronting academic health centers, should nevertheless be carried out in a manner that supports rather than harms the valued social missions of these institutions. Regulation that preserves patient access to the services of the academic center, and that promotes adequate reimbursement for the sicker, more complex mix of patients seen at teaching institutions, would be particularly helpful to academic health centers as they struggle to sustain their missions through a difficult transition of health-care financing and delivery.

REFERENCES

Association of American Medical Colleges (AAMC). 1993. *Academic Medicine and Health Care Reform: Health-Related Research.* Washington, D.C.: AAMC. July.
————. 1996a. *What Americans Say About the Nation's Medical Schools and Teaching Hospitals: Final Report on Public Opinion Research.* Washington, D.C.: AAMC.

————. 1996b. *The Financing of Medical Schools: A Report of the AAMC Task Force on Medical School Financing.* Washington, D.C.: AAMC. November.

————. 1997. *AAMC Fact Sheet.* Vol. 1, no. 7, *Growth in Uncompensated Care Costs in Integrated Academic Medical Centers, 1991–1995.* Washington, D.C.: AAMC. March 3.

————. 1998a. AAMC. *Tomorrow's Doctors, Tomorrow's Cures, The Special Contributions of America's Medical Schools and Teaching Hospitals to the Nation's Health.* Washington, D.C.: AAMC. March. (http://www.aamc.org/about/progemph/tdtc /factshts/special.htm)

————. 1998b. *AAMC Fact Sheet.* Vol. 2, no. 7, *Partnerships for Education between Medical Schools and Managed Care Organizations: The Experience of the University of Connecticut School of Medicine.* Washington, D.C.: AAMC. June.

————. 1998c. *AAMC Issue Briefs. Clinical Research.* Washington, D.C.: AAMC. October 10. (http://www.aamc.org/advocacy/issues/research/clinres.htm)

————. 1998d. *Meeting the Needs of the Community: How Medical Schools and Teaching Hospitals Ensure Access to Clinical Services.* Washington, D.C.: AAMC.

————. 1998e. *AAMC Press Release.* Washington, D.C.: AAMC. November 10. (http://www.aamc.org/advocacy/issues/research/clinres.htm).

————. 1998f. *Washington Highlights.* Washington, D.C.: AAMC. November 13. (http://www.aamc.org/advocacy/washhigh/98nov13/htm).

————. 1998g. *AAMC Issue Briefs.* Medicare Disproportionate Share (DSH) Payments. Washington, D.C.: AAMC. November 10. (http://www.aamc.org/advocacy/issues /research/clinres.htm)

————. 1999a. *AAMC Fact Sheet.* Vol. 3, no. 3, *NIH Research Funding Remains Stable Across All U.S. Medical Schools.* Washington, D.C.: AAMC. March.

————. 1999b. *AAMC Press Release. AAMC Calls for Restoration of BBA Medicare Cuts To Teaching Hospitals.* Washington, D.C.: AAMC. April 28. (http://www.aamc.org /newsroom/pressrel/990428.html)

————. 1999c. *AAMC Fact Sheet.* Vol. 3, no. 5, *Impact of the Balanced Budget Act of 1997 on Major Teaching Hospitals.* Washington, D.C.: AAMC. May.

————. 1999d. *Academic Medicine: The Cornerstone of the American Health Care System.* Washington, D.C.: AAMC. (http://www.aamc.org/hlthcare/start.htm)

————. 1999e. *Press Release.* "AAMC calls for Restoration of BBA Medicare Cuts to Teaching Hospitals." Washington, D.C.: AAMC. April 28. (www.aamc.org /news room/pressrel/chron.htm).

————. 2000. *Issue Briefs. America's Teaching Hospitals Still Hurt from the BBA.* Washington, D.C.: AAMC. April 26. (http://www.aamc.org/advocacy/issues/medicare /ibba.htm)

Biles, B. 1997. *Briefing Note: Changes in Medicare Payments to Academic Health Centers Help Level the Playing Field.* New York: Commonwealth Fund. November.

Biles, B., and L. Simon. 1996. "Academic Health Centers in an Era of Managed Care." *Bulletin of the New York Academy of Medicine* 63:485–89.

Blake, D. A. 1996. "Commentary: Whither Academic Values during the Transition from Academic Medical Center to Integrated Health Delivery Systems?" *Acad. Med.* 71 (8): 818–19.

Blumenthal, D. 1998. Presentation to the Annual Meeting of the Association of American Medical Colleges, Center for the Assessment and Management of Change in Academic Medicine Session. New Orleans. October.

Blumenthal, D., E. G. Campbell, and J. S. Weissman. 1997. "The Social Missions of Academic Health Centers." Sounding Board. *New Eng. J. Med.* 337(21): 1550–53.

Blumenthal, D., and G. Meyer. 1995. "The Response of Academic Health Centers to Health Care Reform." In *Academic Health Centers in the Managed Care Environment,* ed. D. Korn, C. McLaughlin, and M. Osterweis. Washington, D.C.: Association of Academic Health Centers.

————. 1996. "Academic Health Centers in a Changing Environment." *Health Affairs* 15(2): 201–15.

Blumenthal, D., and S. O. Thier. 1998. "Leveling the Playing Field: A Report of the Commonwealth Fund Task Force on Academic Health Centers." (Review). *J. Urban Health* 75(2):330–46.

Brody, H., and V. L. Bonham, Jr. 1997. "Gag Rules and Trade Secrets in Managed Care Contracts: Ethical and Legal Concerns." *Archives of Internal Medicine* 157:2037–43.

Carey, R. M., and C. L. Engelhard. 1996. "Academic Medicine Meets Managed Care: A High-Impact Collision." *Acad. Med.* 71(8): 839–45.

Carli, T. 1999. "The Washtenaw Integrated Healthcare Project." *Washtenaw County Medical Society Bulletin* 50(5): 9–10.

Cerra, F. B. 1997. "Frank B. Cerra, M.D." Interview. *Journal of Investigative Medicine* 45 (8): 416–22.

Cohen, J. J. 1996. "Clinical Research is a Damsel in Distress." *Acad. Med.* 7(9): 984.

Commonwealth Task Force on Academic Health Centers. 1997. *Leveling the Playing Field: Financing the Missions of Academic Health Centers.* New York: Commonwealth Fund.

————. 1998. *Report of the Commonwealth Foundation's Task Force on Academic Health Centers.* New York: Commonwealth Fund.

Cyphert, S. T., J. W. Colloton, and S. Levey. 1997. "Academic Health Center Teaching Hospitals in Transition: A Perspective from the Field." *Best Practices and Benchmarking in Healthcare* 6:258–64.

Dobson, A., K. Coleman, and R. Mechanic. 1994. *Analysis of Teaching Hospital Costs.* Fairfax, Va.: Lewin-VHI.

Foreman S. 1994. "Statement on Academic Medicine in an Era of Health Care Reform." Testimony of the Association of American Medical Colleges, presented April 14 before the Committee on Finance, U.S. Senate, Washington, D.C.

Gold, M. R. 1996. "Effects of the Growth of Managed Care on Academic Medical Centers and Graduate Medical Education." *Acad. Med.* 71(8): 828–38.

Griner, P. F. 1998. "Introduction." In *Meeting the Needs of the Community: How Medical Schools and Teaching Hospitals Ensure Access to Clinical Services.* Washington, D.C.: AAMC.

Griner, P. F., and D. Blumenthal. 1998. "Reforming the Structure and Management of Academic Medical Centers: Case Studies of Ten Institutions." *Acad. Med.* 73(7): 818–25.

Hadley, J., and D. J. Gaskin. 1995. "Policy Brief: Preliminary Evidence on the Impact of HMO Enrollment in Academic Health Centers." Washington, D.C.: Institute for Health Care Research and Policy. Unpublished manuscript, December.

Health Care Financing Administration (HCFA). 1998. *Highlights—National Health Expenditures, 1998.* (http://hcfa.gov/stats/nhe-oact/hilites.htm)

Henderson, T. M. 1999. *Funding of Graduate Medical Education by State Medicaid Programs.* Washington, D.C.: Association of American Medical Colleges. April.

Himmelstein, D. U., and S. Woolhandler. 1997. "Bound to Gag." *Archives of Internal Medicine* 157(18): 2033 (Oct. 13).

Iezzoni, L. I., J. Z. Ayanian, D. W. Bates, and H. R. Burstin. 1998. "Paying More Fairly for Medicare Capitated Care." *New Eng. J. Med.* 339:1933–38.

Iglehart, J. K. 1994. "The American Health Care System—Teaching Hospitals." *New Eng. J. Med.* 329(14): 1052–56.

———. 1999a. "The American Health Care System—Medicare." *New Eng. J. Med.* 340 (4): 327–32 (Jan.).

———. 1999b. "The American Health Care System—Medicaid." *New Eng. J. Med.* 340 (5): 403–8 (Feb.).

Jones, R. F., and S. C. Sanderson. 1996. "Clinical Revenues Used to Support the Academic Mission of Medical Schools, 1992–1993." *Acad. Med.* 71:299–307.

Kassirer, J. P. 1994. "Academic Medical Centers Under Siege." Editorial. *New Eng. J. Med.* 331(20): 1370–71.

Kirschner, M. W., E. Marincola, and E. O. Taisberg. 1994. "The Role of Biomedical Research in Health Care Reform." *Science* 266:49–51.

Localio, A. R., A. G. Lawthers, T. A. Brennan, N. M. Laird, L. E. Hebert, L. M. Peterson, J. P. Newhouse, P. C. Weiler, and H. H. Hiatt. 1991. "Relation between Malpractice Claims and Adverse Events Due to Negligence: Results of the Harvard Medical Practice Study III." *New Eng. J. Med.* 325:245–51.

Lurie, N. 1996. "Preparing Physicians for Practice in Managed Care Environments." *Acad. Med.* 71(10): 1044–49.

Mechanic, D., and M. Schlesinger. 1996. "The Impact of Managed Care on Patients' Trust in Medical Care and Their Physicians." *JAMA* 275(21): 1693–97 (June 5).

Mechanic, R. E., and A. Dobson. 1996. "The Impact of Managed Care on Clinical Research: A Preliminary Investigation." *Health Affairs* 15(3): 72–89.

Moore, G. T. 1993. *Report to the Council on Graduate Medical Education.* Washington, D.C.: COGME.

Moy, E. 1998a. "Care of Medically Underserved Patients by Teaching Hospitals." In *Meeting the Needs of the Community: How Medical Schools and Teaching Hospitals Ensure Access to Clinical Services.* Washington, D.C.: AAMC.

———. 1998b. "Care of the Severely Ill: Variations in Case-Mix between Teaching and Other Hospitals." In *Meeting the Needs of the Community: How Medical Schools and Teaching Hospitals Ensure Access to Clinical Services.* Washington, D.C.: AAMC.

Moy, E., A. J. Mazzaschi, R. J. Levin, D. A. Blake, and P. F. Griner. 1997. "Relationship between National Institutes of Health Research Awards to U.S. Medical Schools and Managed Care Market Penetration." *JAMA* 278(3): 217–21.

Moy, E., E. Valente, R. J. Levin, K. J. Bhak, and P. F. Griner. 1996a. "Academic Medical Centers and the Care of Underserved Populations." *Acad. Med.* 71(12): 1370–77.

———. 1996b. "The Volume and Mix of Inpatient Services Provided by Academic Medical Centers." *Acad. Med.* 71(10): 1116–22 (October).

Pardes, H. 1997. "The Future of Medical Schools and Teaching Hospitals in the Era of Managed Care." *Acad. Med.* 72(2): 97–102.

Physician Payment Review Commission. 1994. *Annual Report to Congress, 1994.* Washington, D.C.: PPRC.

Relman, A. S. 1992. "'Self-Referral'—What's at Stake?" *New Eng. J. Med.* 327(21): 1522–24.

Reuter, J. A. 1997. *The Balanced Budget Act of 1997: Implications for Medical Education.*

Task Force on Academic Health Centers. New York: Commonwealth Fund. October.

Reuter, J., D. Gaskin, and J. Hadley. 1996. *HMOs' Use of Academic Centers.* Washington, D.C.: Institute for Health Care Research and Policy, Georgetown University. March.

Rodwin, M. A. 1995. "Conflicts in Managed Care." *New Eng. J. Med.* 332(9): 604–7.

Sinaiko, R. 1996. "Academic Medical Centers and Managed Care: Adapting to a Changing Health Care Marketplace." In *Managed Care Perspectives,* supplement to *Managed Care Week.* Washington, D.C.: Atlantic Information Services. September 30.

"Teaching Hospitals in Trouble." 1999. Editorial. *New York Times,* May 31, p. A18.

U.S. General Accounting Office. 1997. "Managed Care: Explicit Gag Clauses Not Found in HMO Contracts, But Physicians' Concerns Remain." GAO/HEHS-97-175. Washington, D.C.: U.S. Government Printing Office.

Valente, E., and K. G. Serrin. 1998. "Uncompensated Care in Major Teaching Hospitals and Faculty Practice Plans." In *Meeting the Needs of the Community: How Medical Schools and Teaching Hospitals Ensure Access to Clinical Services.* Washington, D.C.: AAMC.

Weissman, J. S., D. Saglam, E. G. Campbell, N. Causino, and D. Blumenthal. 1999. "Market Forces and Unsponsored Research in Academic Health Centers." *JAMA* 281(12): 1093–98.

Woolhandler, S., and D. U. Himmelstein. 1995. "Extreme Risk—The New Corporate Proposition for Physicians." *New Eng. J. Med.* 333(25): 1706–8.

PART 3

Purchasers and Market Oversight

CHAPTER 7

Markets for Medicine?

Keith J. Crocker and John R. Moran

> Lawyers for a South Scranton woman have filed a lawsuit alleging a doctor caused her husband's death by denying the man access to needed emergency health care. Attorneys for Joyce Cerep are filing a civil suit . . . alleging that [the doctor] refused treatment to her late husband James in order to save money. . . . According to the suit, 33-year old James Cerep died in 1994 from lack of oxygen because of a seizure he suffered in his bathroom. Joyce Cerep allegedly called [the doctor] several times for authorization to call an ambulance and get help for her husband. "[The doctor] told Joyce Cerep he did not feel this was a medical emergency and she should wait at least half an hour before calling for help," said [the wife's attorney].
>
> —*Scranton Times*, April 15, 1996

The introduction of economic incentives in the provision of health-care services through the use of managed care has generated a substantial amount of controversy, in part because of a proliferation of anecdotes alleging systematic underprovision of care. Judging from the debate in the public press, it might appear that, in moving from fee-for-service arrangements to managed care, we have simply traded one problem for another. A common argument against the traditional fee-for-service system—and, by implication, for support of the managed-care alternative—is that the incentives inherent in the arrangement virtually guarantee that health care will be overprovided. The patients do not know what is wrong with them and rely on health-care providers to diagnose and treat their afflictions. And, since the health-care providers are compensated by the insurers for the treatments provided, they have every reason to err on the side of making sure that no diagnostic stone is left unturned. Finally, the health-care insurer is simply left to foot the bill and compensates for the overtreatment by charging higher premiums to all consumers.

An unfortunate result of the perception that fee-for-service arrangements overprovide, and managed care underprovides, has been the increasingly common assertion that medical care is somehow beyond the pale when it comes to economic analysis (see, for example, Rice 1997). According to this line of thought, there is something *unique* about heath care that makes the application of standard economic arguments inappropriate. While we recognize that there may be noneconomic or ethical concerns that could be used to argue for the use of nonmarket mechanisms in the provision of health care, our goal in this chapter is to deal with the economic issues.

A Thought Experiment

It would perhaps be useful to consider for a moment the proposition that the particulars of the institutional and informational environment endemic to health care would make this an area uniquely unqualified to the use of the market mechanism. As we have already discussed, the difficulties in the traditional fee-for-service provision of health care are argued to arise from a confluence of conflicting incentives: patients do not know what is wrong with them, they just want to be cured, and they do not care about the cost; providers know what the patients need and, since they are reimbursed by the insurer for the treatment expenses incurred, may find it profitable to overprescribe treatment; and, finally, insurers rely on the providers' diagnoses and simply pay the bill. Moreover, these tendencies are amplified by the burgeoning problems of malpractice liability, which has made the overtreatment option even more attractive to providers, since it is then easier to argue that they have performed their duties scrupulously.

These conditions are, however, less unique than commonly supposed. In order to focus our intuition on these issues, let us consider an alternative, and somewhat more mundane, insurance setting: the purchase of collision insurance for automobiles. When faced with property damage to an automobile, the owner simply desires to have the car repaired and returned to its original serviceable condition. Few automobile owners have the ability to ascertain the nature of the necessary repairs and so rely heavily on the expertise of the body repair shop operator, who is in this case the provider of (repair) services. In a setting where the automobile is fixed by an independent body shop, there clearly are incentives to engage in overrepair, which could be a unilaterally profitable strategy by the body shop involving unnecessary repairs with inflated bills, or it could involve the assent of the owner through, say, the repair of earlier (uninsured) damage or other improvements to the car. In addition, the insurer relies on the diagnosis of the repair shops and pays the resulting bill. As a consequence, in many instructive ways, this market would seem to suffer the same types of informational and incentive problems, with the consequence of service overprovision by the provider, that would appear to characterize the market for health-care services.

There are, of course, mechanisms that have arisen in this market whose purpose is to mitigate these incentive problems. In the event of a claim for accident damage, some insurers send out a claims adjuster—who may be either an employee of the insurer or an independent agent—to examine the extent of the damage and to negotiate with the provider of repair services over the nature and costs of the repairs to be performed. Other insurers adopt a less intrusive posture and merely require the owner of the automobile to obtain, for example, three estimates for repair from different body shops and then direct that the shop providing the lowest estimate be used. Finally, some insurers do not intrude at all on the owner's decisions regarding repair and simply pay the repair bill submitted by the shop that was selected by the owner to perform the repairs. Not surprisingly, the result has been a somewhat bifurcated insurance market, where consumers have the choice either of purchasing inexpensive collision coverage, which is generally associated with substantial restrictions on the choice of repair providers available to the insured, or of obtaining a more expensive policy, but one that permits broader consumer choice when it comes to the selection of a service provider.

While there are intriguing similarities between collision and health-care insurance, there are, of course, also substantial and qualitative differences. Perhaps one of the most instructive differences is the nature of the coverage being provided: whereas collision insurance does not apply to routine maintenance and related expenditures required to keep the car in working order, health insurance is designed to indemnify patients against routine illnesses and, in many cases, fairly predictable afflictions. Put differently, automobile insurance never covers valve jobs, but health insurance does. Why the difference, and what are the ramifications?

The traditional argument for the lack of insurance for automobile maintenance costs has centered around the economic problem of "moral hazard"— that, once afforded the protection provided by such insurance, the owner would not have any incentive to take care of the car, which would increase the chances of the insured-upon hazard occurring. For example, why bother to incur the expense of changing the oil when the insurance will repair the resulting engine damage? This type of reasoning has less punch in the case of personal decisions regarding health care. The decision to smoke notwithstanding, most individuals find poor health outcomes, even with insurance, to be fairly unpleasant, which would seem to mitigate individuals' incentives to act in a way that increases the probability or severity of illness.

Instead, moral hazard in health insurance generally takes the form of greater utilization of health services on the part of insured individuals than would be the case if patients bore the full cost of their care. The reduced price paid at the time service is delivered encourages insureds to use the system with both greater frequency (by, for example, seeking treatment for minor or transitory ailments) and greater intensity (as when more efficacious or convenient treatments are substituted for less costly alternatives).

Another important distinction between the two types of coverage is the lack of an objective, agreed-upon upper bound on the value of many medical interventions. In the case of auto insurance, the potential cost to the insurer is limited by the value of a repair, which is in turn bounded by the cost of replacing the automobile. When accidents result in severe damage, insurers can opt to limit their liability to the current "blue book" value of the automobile, without adversely affecting the degree of loss protection conferred on the insured. This is in marked contrast to health insurance, where lifetime benefit caps and other coverage limitations (such as restrictions on coverage for experimental treatments) significantly increase the loss exposure of insureds and, in some cases, may limit their access to potentially lifesaving treatments. This problem is further exacerbated by the large, technology-driven variability in aggregate health-care costs, which creates a source of undiversifiable risk for health insurers and further limits the extent to which medical care can be insured (Cutler 1993).

Managed Care: A Panacea?

A primary economic argument for replacing a fee-for-service arrangement with a managed-care relationship is that, by doing so, the insurer can obtain direct control over the providers, thereby mitigating the problem of service overprovision. The degree and type of influence that managed-care plans exert over physicians vary widely, but virtually all managed-care organizations attempt to integrate cost considerations into physician decision making in one way or another. In some cases, this involves selective recruiting of physicians who have cultivated a cost-conscious practice style. Although information on physician practice styles is typically obtained informally, a number of plans have recently begun using quantitative information on the patterns of care exhibited by area doctors, a practice commonly known as "profiling." A case in point is the development of the "Pro/File" computer system, which has been used by a number of managed-care plans to track physicians' use of resources, both over time and on a per-patient or per-illness basis. The system also provides information on how frequently physicians order diagnostic tests and how often they refer patients to specialists (Goldstein 1992). Ratings of physicians generated by this system were used by Blue Cross Blue Shield of the National Capital Area as the basis for a solicitation of nearly three thousand area doctors to join a new managed-care network (Iglehart 1992).

In addition to seeking doctors with an interest in cost-effective medicine, managed-care organizations also use a variety of rules and incentives to promote cost control. In their study of physicians' arrangements with managed-care plans, Gold et al. (1995) found that almost all HMOs have some form of utilization review (such as preadmission review for hospital admissions, discharge planning, and ambulatory review for resource-intensive services) and that about three-quarters also have formal practice guidelines that designate which treatments and tests are medically appropriate under various clinical conditions. Perhaps of more direct concern to the patient, over 80 percent of managed-care plans require patients to select a primary care physician, to whom they must go for referrals to specialists (Gold et al. 1995).

Physicians in managed-care organizations also face a number of pecuniary incentives to economize on the provision of services. The most prominent among these are payment adjustments based on utilization or cost measures (57 percent of plans) and physician risk sharing, sometimes in the form of capitation, in which some portion of the physician's revenue or income is based on the difference between the amount spent on each patient and a fixed per-patient payment made to the physician at the beginning of each month (60 percent of plans). As of 1994, 37 percent of managed-care plans were using capitation as the predominant method of paying primary care physicians (Gold et al. 1995). Moreover, the use of risk sharing as part of physician compensation for services is also on the rise among nonprofit HMOs, including the well-known Fallon Community Health Plan and the Kaiser Foundation Health Plans (Gabel 1997). Perhaps the single most important incentive that many doctors face is the (implicit) threat that they will be dropped from the plan's panel if their practice style is viewed as extravagant. While little direct evidence is available on this point, it stands to reason that deselection is a potentially powerful sanction, particularly in small communities, where a large proportion of a provider's prospective patients belongs to the plan in question.

While these mechanisms may certainly serve to reduce the incentives of providers to overprovide health-care services, another problem is introduced as a result. Patients still rely on the providers to diagnose treatments, but now the incentive may well be for *underprovision* of services by the providers whose incentives are being shaped by the pressures for cost minimization emanating from the insurance payer. The key question, of course, is this: do providers respond to these incentives and, if so, to what extent is patient care compromised? Although little is known about the impact on patient outcomes, available evidence suggests that providers *do* respond to the types of financial incentives commonly employed by managed-care plans (Hillman 1987; Hillman, Pauly, and Kerstein 1989). And, interestingly enough, there does seem to be a perception among consumers that this may indeed be the case, as evidenced by the increased popularity of products such as point-of-service plans that permit the insured to opt out of the strictures of the managed-care plan, albeit at the cost of higher up-front insurance premiums and larger copayments.

The issue of whether the reduction in resource use stemming from physician financial incentives results in the withholding of *needed* care is the subject of ongoing debate. Early studies did not detect significant differences in patient outcomes across managed-care and fee-for-service systems (Miller and Luft 1994). The conclusions from these studies must be viewed with caution, however, due to the small number of plans studied and their focus on a time period when competition and incentives for cost containment were less acute than they are today (Luft 1988). A more recent analysis that followed 2,235 patients over a four-year period found that elderly and poor patients with chronic medical conditions had worse outcomes when enrolled in HMOs than when covered by fee-for-service insurance (Ware et al. 1996).

Restrictive practices have also been implicated, anecdotally, in a number of instances in which patients have suffered grievous harm. Since these stories are so numerous and extensively documented in the popular press, we need not dwell on them here. But, as these types of examples suggest, there are two obvious avenues by which health-care services might be underprovided in a managed-care setting. The first occurs when an individual signs up for a plan without a full understanding of what is and is not covered by the agreement. A common source of conflict occurs when a patient discovers that a "state-of-the-art" treatment for an affliction, such as bone marrow transplantation for breast cancer, is not covered because it is deemed to be "experimental" by the managed-care plan. These types of misunderstandings regarding coverage are, unfortunately, not all that uncommon in insurance agreements generally and undoubtedly serve as a source of substantial income for professional litigators. This problem is particularly pronounced in the health-care sector because health care is unlike most insurance settings, in which claims occur only in the rare event of an accident or other calamity. In health care, payments are made on behalf of insured individuals to health-care providers on a regular basis. Moreover, the range of potentially covered afflictions and treatments is certainly beyond the scope of understanding for a typical insured, such that the possibilities for either stealth exclusions or more affirmative acts of skulduggery are enhanced.

A second source of underprovision is more insidious and arises from the fact that the provider (who, as discussed earlier, is also the payer in the case of many managed-care plans) provides the diagnosis and treatment and the patient relies on the provider's judgment in this regard. In many cases, a patient who is denied a particular, and costly, course of treatment in favor of a less expensive alternative never knows that she or he has been less than fully treated by the health-care provider. And, the proliferation of gag clauses that prohibit providers from discussing treatment options certainly serves to exacerbate this problem.

In response to the increasing concerns about the potential for managed care to result in the underprovision of health care, several changes to the current system have been advocated.

Setting a Minimum Standard

The suggestion that the services provided by managed-care providers should be regulated at either the state or the federal level has become increasingly popular as the various horror story anecdotes involving withheld care have circulated. This view has been evidenced most recently by the extensive support in some political circles for a Patients' Bill of Rights, whose purpose would be to circumscribe the providers' abilities to withhold care. The particulars of the various proposals vary, but most seem to include the following types of provisions.

- Prohibiting gag clauses that penalize doctors for referring to specialists or for revealing to their patients the existence of more costly medical treatments.
- Prohibiting managed-care plans from rewarding doctors who restrict their patients' access to expensive procedures.
- Requiring plans to offer medically necessary treatments, if the procedure is consistent with the accepted principles of practice.

The proponents of such reforms argue that these changes would put patients on a more level playing field in their relationship with their managed-care provider, resulting in a fairer and more efficacious course of treatment.

As a first cut, it would seem that an easy solution to the problem of the underprovision of care would be simply to mandate higher levels of care, with appropriate penalties for noncompliant providers. A primary difficulty with this approach, however, revolves around the issue of the level at which these mandated services should be set. If the standards are set too high, then the resulting premiums may cause lower-income individuals to be priced out of the market and may leave them with the prospect of going without health-care coverage. A "crowd out" effect of this variety has been implicated in the low rate of health insurance provision among small employers, although the available evidence on the magnitude of the effect has been mixed (Jensen and Gabel 1992; Gruber 1994). Moreover, it could be argued that even those with higher incomes may be disadvantaged, as it may well be the case that many who could afford the plan with mandated benefits would, instead, *prefer* to purchase a lower level of services but would be precluded from doing so because of the minimum standards imposed by regulation.

The need to guarantee affordability of a mandated plan would likely require that the minimum standards be set at relatively low levels, which may well serve to eliminate some of the more egregious examples of service underprovision. But, such a minimalist approach does not help the purchasers of plans that exceed the minimum standards to sort between the competing alternatives.

Providing Clear Statements of Coverages and Limitations

A concern often voiced by those unhappy with their managed-care plans is the existence of limitations or exclusions in the plans' coverages that were not anticipated by the consumers at the time they chose their health-care providers. Part of the problem, of course, is that health care is a remarkably complex and technologically evolving product whose multidimensional attributes exceed the analytic abilities of even the most discerning and capable consumer. Add to this a mind-numbing range of potential treatment options whose relative advantages in terms of costs or efficacy are at best vaguely understood by the average person, and we have a market where effective comparison shopping by consumers may be difficult.

One possibility would be to effect a regulatory requirement that the plans clearly and accurately reveal the nature of the exclusions they contain, as well as indicate the fashion in which their providers are compensated and any restrictions (such as gag clauses) on the doctors regarding either the treatment or the information they may provide to patients. While most consumers can ascertain the particulars of coverage in many insurance settings where the trade-offs are more obvious and concrete (for example, damage to a car from a break-in may be covered but not the laptop computer stolen off the car's seat), in many cases determining the appropriate type of treatment is more problematical, even among health-care professionals. Determining what is and is not covered by a particular plan requires not only an examination of the particulars of the formal managed-care contract but also an examination of how specific situations have been interpreted, and the nature of the treatments approved, by the managed-care plan in the past. Thus, attempts to codify the coverages of competing managed-care plans in a formulaic manner that permits consumers to make unambiguous comparisons between the attributes offered promises to be a daunting, if not impossible, task.

In addition to understanding the coverage limitations specified under each plan, consumers must also gauge the overall quality of care that they are likely to receive from plan providers. In the case of medical services, "quality of care" can be thought of as encompassing both technical quality, which refers to the expertise of providers in diagnosing and treating illness, and nontechnical quality, which refers to the more mundane aspects of care, such as waiting times, the ease with which appointments can be made, and the general attentiveness of doctors and staff (Wyszewianski 1988). Consumers' widely recognized inability to judge the technical aspects of quality is especially problematic in an era of managed care, where choice of a health plan often entails precommitment to a particular set of providers for periods of up to a year.

One attempt to deal with this problem has been the use of "health plan report cards" to help consumers sort through the differences between competing managed-care plans. Beginning in the late 1980s, several large employers and managed-care organizations combined to develop a set of standardized performance measures, known as the Health Plan Employer Data and Information Set, that could be used to make comparative judgments about the overall performance of health plans (Custer 1995). The HEDIS measures, which include information on patient satisfaction, cost and utilization of services, and the availability of preventive care, form the backbone of many report cards in use today.

Although surveys consistently show that consumers want more information on plans and providers, several recent studies indicate that the current generation of performance measures may not be particularly helpful. For example, Robinson and Brodie (1997) report that only 34 percent of consumers who have access to standardized performance ratings report having used them in their decision making. This conclusion is reinforced by a study of actual plan choices in a Fortune 100 company, which found that employees' choices were largely independent of five widely used performance measures enumerated in a company-sponsored report card (Chernew and Scanlon 1998). The authors conjecture that the lack of a systematic relationship between plan choices and report card ratings could reflect either the superiority of the information already possessed by consumers or the inherent conflicts in how certain aspects of plan performance were evaluated. For example, the measure of surgical care used in their study presumes that higher utilization of various surgeries, such as coronary artery bypass surgery or cardiac catheterization, is a *negative* attribute of the plan, such that plans that perform more of these procedures score *lower* in the ratings. While such a judgment may accord well with the preferences of cost-conscious employers, it should not be surprising that performing fewer of these state-of-the-art procedures may be viewed as a red flag by consumers concerned about utilization controls (Chernew and Scanlon 1998). Of course, a system that rated plans favorably simply for having performed large numbers of these surgeries may be even less desirable.

A similar problem arises when using measures based on patient satisfaction. In their study, Chernew and Scanlon (1998) found that plans with higher patient satisfaction ratings had *lower* enrollments, all other things equal. They speculate that this may be due to longer waiting periods and fewer physicians accepting new patients in plans employing the most sought-after doctors. Such conflicts over how the quality of care is best judged are not new and point to the numerous difficulties that must be confronted in constructing useful ratings of plan performance. Nevertheless, as HEDIS continues to be refined and is expanded to include measures of patient outcomes, it hopefully will evolve into a more useful tool for assessing the merits of competing health plans. Such better information on health plan performance may help consumers and employers cure this "market imperfection," thereby allowing market forces to reward high-quality and efficient providers.

A more intrusive regulatory approach to this market imperfection, but one that has some attractiveness from the perspective of transparency, would be to implement a scheme of the type currently used in the Medigap market to provide supplementary coverage for Medicare beneficiaries. Motivated in large part by perceptions of improprieties in the Medigap market Congress enacted legislation in 1980 (P.L. 96–265) that established requirements for policies that were advertised as "Medicare supplements." Although these policies included the required information on minimum benefits and plan attributes to be provided to potential purchasers, consumers were still left with the task of sorting out the particulars of the various, and disparate, plans that cleared the regulatory hurdle. To further reduce the burden consumers faced in comparing alternative Medigap plans, Congress in 1990 revised the regulation of Medicare supplements, with the result that plans were restricted to a menu of ten preapproved benefits packages. This standardization of permitted Medigap plans, while reducing somewhat the spectrum of consumer choices, certainly increased the ability of purchasers to understand the nature of what they were purchasing and facilitated comparison shopping (Rice, Graham, and Fox 1997).

A similar strategy might be implemented in the context of managed-care plans in an attempt to reduce the informational disadvantage that purchasers face when considering the attributes of alternative managed-care plans. In such a setting, consumers could use the ordinal ranking provided by a standardized menu of plans to select a level of health-care coverage that accorded with their own health-care needs and financial circumstances. Since plans within each permitted category would be homogenous in terms of the services offered, price competition between the providers would be enhanced. And, since the various levels of coverage would be designed by the regulatory authority, the categories could be crafted in a fashion that permitted meaningful comparisons by consumers across the types of plans.

A Few More—Exotic—Possibilities

One undoubtedly controversial approach to mitigate any problems pertaining to the underprovision of health care would be to unleash the tort system and to permit patients who are injured by the withholding of treatment to sue their managed-care plan. As Peter Jacobson notes in chapter 13, some courts have interpreted ERISA to exempt certain employer-based benefit plans—including ERISA-covered managed-care plans—from any state laws regarding malpractice. The effect of this ERISA preemption is to shield such managed-care plans from legal claims demanding compensation by patients for losses suffered as a result of the treatment received or not received.

While few observers would dispute the fact that the tort system—with the usual visions of ambulance-chasing attorneys and endless litigation—has substantial, and costly, shortcomings, it is also equally clear that the lingering threat of a malpractice claim can make the withholding of treatment by a managed-care provider a less economic, and therefore less attractive, strategy. But, given the state of employee benefits law, the ability to discipline recalcitrant managed-care providers by using the club of tort enforcement is strictly circumscribed, absent either a statutory change in the wording of the law or a reinterpretation by the courts of the law as it currently stands.

An alternative approach for dealing with the underprovision of health services under managed care would be to return to a more traditional fee-for-service system, but one in which individuals were required to self-insure against small losses while at the same time receiving relatively complete protection against more catastrophic events. Such "major risk" health insurance would avoid the incentives for underprovision inherent in managed care, while mitigating, at least partially, the propensity of insured individuals to overconsume health-care services. A typical major risk policy would specify a 50 percent coinsurance rate for all medical care up to an out-of-pocket limit of 10 percent of the insured's income. Above the limit, all care would be fully insured.

It has been estimated that widespread adoption of this type of policy would reduce aggregate health-care spending by approximately 20 percent, with the largest reductions concentrated among high-income persons (Feldstein and Gruber 1994). Proponents argue that a major risk policy could be provided to every person under the age of sixty-five at a monthly premium of approximately $150 per person if the tax deductibility of employer-paid health insurance premiums was eliminated. Alternatively, individuals might be induced to voluntarily purchase a major risk plan if out-of-pocket medical expenditures were made tax deductible or if medical expenses could be funded with pretax dollars through a medical savings account.

The principal appeal of the major risk approach is that, by incentivizing patients rather than providers, overprovision of services can be substantially reduced without "managing" patient care through the kinds of physician financial incentives and restrictions on provider choice that consumers find so odious. A potential problem with the major risk approach is that such policies may appeal primarily to healthier members of the population, leaving those with higher medical expenses in more comprehensive plans. This, in turn, would force high-end plans to increase their premiums, potentially resulting in a "death spiral" in which plans providing more comprehensive coverage are driven from the market. While this type of arrangement has yet to be tried on a large scale, recent attempts to market medical savings accounts through a congressionally mandated pilot program have apparently failed to generate much interest on the part of consumers. If not universal and mandated, such medical savings account options could be selected preferentially by the healthy, leaving the expensive unhealthy population in the full coverage plan, further driving costs of these plans upward.

Finally, an intriguing and thought-provoking alternative to managed care has been suggested by Robin Hanson (1994), who notes that one of the shortcomings of traditional health-care plans is that they are concerned with the provision of *health-care services,* while the truly important issue to the patient is the *health outcome.* As a consequence, the debate has focused on the level of services provided by either fee-for-service (often too much) or managed-care (arguably too little) plans rather than on the incentives of the health-care provider to keep the patient *healthy.* Hanson argues that one way of dealing with the problem of getting the health-care provider to supply the correct amount and type of health care is to put the provider in a position where she or he is concerned with the health of the patient rather than with the cost of providing treatment. One way to accomplish this would be to have the patient purchase a *combination* life insurance and health-care plan. So, for a single premium, the health-care provider would promise to provide both health care for the insured as well as a stipulated death benefit of, say, *x* amount of dollars.

The effect of instituting this hypothetical plan would be to change dramatically the incentives of the provider to keep the consumer healthy, particularly if the insured chooses to purchase a policy with a large face value. In contrast to the current situation, where, after the premiums have been collected every dollar spent on treatment is a dollar less in profit for the health-care provider, the hybrid plan makes investments by the provider in health care more attractive since such expenditures reduce the likelihood of having to pay the death benefit. Put differently, in such a setting, providing care would no longer be a pure cost to the provider but, rather, would become a potential profit center. Such plans, however, might encourage inappropriate prolongation of care past the point of a patient's choice to desist. Also, it might discourage doctors from accepting or keeping the more seriously ill patient.

Will Managed Care Reduce the Growth in Health-Care Costs?

As managed-care penetration grew rapidly in the early 1990s, it was hoped that managed care would play a role in restraining the growth in overall health-care costs, which, at the time, were rising at alarming levels. These hopes were buttressed by early successes among managed-care organizations in reducing expenditures below the levels typically observed under conventional fee-for-service insurance. Unfortunately, these reductions in the *level* of expenditures have not been matched by corresponding reductions in the *growth* of expenditures, as recent studies have found that total spending is rising at similar rates in managed-care plans as it is in traditional indemnity plans (Newhouse 1993).

In attempting to understand this phenomenon, researchers have focused on two possible explanations. The first is that health maintenance organizations may have initially benefitted from favorable risk selection, due to an unwillingness on the part of older individuals and those with chronic medical conditions to enroll in plans that restricted their choice of physicians and specialists (Hellinger 1995). Thus, the initial enrollees in health maintenance organizations were likely healthier than were those who remained in fee-for-service plans, leading to lower utilization and expenditures under the former. However, as the prevalence of managed care has grown, enrollees in such plans have necessarily become more representative of the population as a whole in terms of their underlying health status and, consequently, have utilized the system to a greater extent, and at a greater cost, than have their healthier predecessors.

A second explanation highlights the key role played by technological change in driving health-care costs. After much study, many analysts have concluded that the primary determinant of escalating health expenditures is the adoption and diffusion of new medical technologies (Newhouse 1993). Because managed-care insurers, and the hospitals with which they contract, have generally adopted new technologies at similar rates as fee-for-service providers (Chernew and Scanlon 1998), it should not be surprising that the growth in health-care expenditures in managed-care organizations has paralleled growth rates among other insurers.

For these reasons, observers of the health-care system have become increasingly skeptical about the ability of managed care to curtail continued growth in expenditures. Moreover, the backlash again the types of restrictive practices described earlier may result in legislation that further diminishes the ability of managed-care organizations to control utilization and, hence, costs.

Conclusions

There is an inescapable trade-off between the desire to insure oneself against the financial consequences of random fluctuations in one's health and the overconsumption of medical care that results when insured individuals face out-of-pocket prices that are below the cost of the care sought. One (partial) solution to this problem is to use coinsurance to raise the price paid by insureds to levels that efficiently trade off the gains from greater risk sharing against the costs of overuse. If patients had the ability to self-diagnose their ailments, and had a complete understanding of the availability and efficacy of all potential treatments, then coinsurance, by itself, would be sufficient to guarantee an efficient outcome. However, because patients generally do not have this capability, and instead must rely on a physician for diagnosis and treatment, an additional complication is introduced. If payments to doctors are tied to the amount of care provided, as is the case under conventional fee-for-service insurance, then physicians have an incentive to exploit their informational advantage to provide excessive amounts of care. Conversely, if doctors are paid a fixed fee per patient that they must use to cover all medical expenses incurred on the patient's behalf, as is the case under many managed-care plans, then they face incentives to underprovide care and possibly to withhold needed treatments. This three-cornered moral hazard problem, involving the doctor, the patient, and a third-party payer, is at the heart of many of the perplexing issues that confront policymakers today.

Although vexing, such a phenomenon is not unique to the market for medical care. Automobile insurance is subject to a similar three-sided incentive problem, yet there is little feeling on the part of the public that there is a crisis in the market for car insurance akin to the one in health care. The incentive problems that have dominated the debate on managed care are not specific to the provision of health-care services but rather reflect common economic problems often encountered in the analysis of markets more generally. The challenge is to recognize that all of the parties involved—the patients, the providers, and the insurers—respond to economic incentives and to apply those insights in an effort to craft health-care arrangements that respect these behavioral realities.

REFERENCES

Chernew, M., R. Hirth, S. Sonnad, R. Ermann, and A. Fendrick. 1998. "Managed Care, Medical Technology, and Health Care Cost Growth: A Review of the Evidence." *Medical Care Research and Review* 55 (September) 3.

Chernew, Michael, and Dennis Scanlon. 1998. "Health Plan Report Cards and Insurance Choice." *Inquiry* 35 (spring): 9–22.

Custer, W. 1995. "Measuring the Quality of Health Care." *Employee Benefit Research Institute Issue Brief* 159 (Mar.): 1–18.

Cutler, David. 1993. "Why Doesn't the Market Fully Insure Long-Term Care?" National Bureau of Economic Research working paper no. 4301. Cambridge: Harvard University. March.

Encinosa, William, and David Sappington. 1997. "Competition among Health Maintenance Organizations." *Journal of Economics and Management Strategy* 7 (spring): 129–50.

Feldstein, Martin, and Jonathan Gruber. 1994. "A Major Risk Approach to Health Insurance Reform." NBER working paper no. 4852. Cambridge: Massachusetts Institute of Technology. September.

Gabel, Jon. 1997. "Ten Ways HMOs Have Changed During the 1990s." *Health Affairs* 16: 134–45.

Gaynor, Martin, and William Vogt. 1997. "What Does Economics Have to Say about Health Policy Anyway?: A Comment and Correction on Evans and Rice." *Journal of Health Politics, Policy, and Law* 22 (Apr.): 475–96.

Gold, Marsha, Robert Hurley, Timothy Lake, Todd Ensor, and Robert Berenson. 1995. "A National Survey of the Arrangements Managed-Care Plans Make with Physicians." *New Eng. J. Med.* 333 (Dec. 21): 1678–83.

Goldstein, A. 1992. "Area Doctors Rated by Cost." *Washington Post,* July 10, p. A1.

Gruber, Jonathan. 1994. "State-Mandated Benefits and Employer-Provided Health Insurance." *Journal of Public Economics* 55:433–64.

Gruber, Jonathan, and Maria Owings. 1996. "Physician Financial Incentives and Cesarean Section Delivery." *Rand Journal of Economics* 27 (spring): 99–123.

Hanson, Robin. 1994. "Buy Health, Not Health Care." *Cato Journal* 14 (spring/summer): 135–41.

Hellinger, Fred. 1995. "Selection Bias in HMOs and PPOs: A Review of the Evidence." *Inquiry* 32:135–42.

Hillman, Alan. 1987. "Financial Incentives for Physicians in HMOs: Is There a Conflict of Interest?" *New Eng. J. Med.* 317 (Dec. 31): 1743–48.

Hillman, Alan, Mark Pauly, and Joseph Kerstein. 1989. "How Do Financial Incentives Affect Physicians' Clinical Decisions and the Financial Performance of Health Maintenance Organizations?" *New Eng. J. Med.* 321 (July 13): 86–92.

Iglehart, John. 1992. "Managed Care." *NEJM* Health Policy Report 327 (Sept. 3): 742–47.

Jensen, Gail, and Jon Gabel. 1992. "State Mandated Benefits and the Small Firm's Decision to Offer Insurance." *Journal of Regulatory Economics* 4:379–404.

Luft, Harold. 1988. "HMOs and the Quality of Care." *Inquiry* 25 (spring): 147–56.

Manning, Willard, Joseph Newhouse, Naihua Duan, Emmett Keeler, Arleen Leibowitz, and Susan Marquis. 1987. "Health Insurance and the Demand for Medical Care: Evidence from a Randomized Experiment." *American Economic Review* 77 (June): 251–77.

Miller, R., and H. Luft. 1994. "Managed Care Plan Performance since 1980: A Literature Analysis." *JAMA* 18 (May): 1512–19.

Moran, Donald. 1997. "Federal Regulation of Managed Care: An Impulse in Search of a Theory." *Health Affairs* 16: 7–21.

Newhouse, Joseph. 1993. "An Iconoclastic View of Health Cost Containment." *Health Affairs* 12 (supplement): 152–71.

Pauly, Mark. 1989. "Taxation, Health Insurance, and Market Failure in the Medical Economy." *Journal of Economic Literature* 24 (June): 629–75.

———. 1997. "Who Was That Straw Man Anyway?: A Comment on Evans and Rice." *Journal of Health Politics, Policy, and Law* 22 (Apr.): 467–73.

Rice, Thomas. 1997. "Can Markets Give Us the Health System We Want?" *Journal of Health Politics, Policy, and Law* 22 (Apr.): 383–426.

Rice, Thomas, Marcia Graham, and Peter Fox. 1997. "The Impact of Policy Standardization on the Medigap Market." *Inquiry* 34 (summer): 106–16.

Robinson, S., and M. Brodie. 1997. "Understanding the Quality Challenge for Health Consumers: The Kaiser/AHCPR Survey." *Journal of Quality Improvement* 23:239–44.

Ware, J., et al. 1996. "Differences in 4-Year Health Outcomes for Elderly and Chronically Ill Patients Treated in HMO and Fee-for-Service Systems." *JAMA* (Oct. 2): 1039–47.

Wyszewianski, L. 1988. "The Emphasis on Measurement in Quality Assurance: Reasons and Implications." *Inquiry* 25 (winter): 424–33.

Zeckhauser, Richard. 1970. "Medical Insurance: A Case Study of the Tradeoff Between Risk Spreading and Appropriate Incentives." *Journal of Economic Theory* 2:10–26.

CHAPTER 8

General Motors as Purchaser

Bruce E. Bradley, James C. Cubbin,
James F. Ball, and Deborah Salerno

The health industry has been under intense pressure to provide high-quality care at low cost.[1] As is evident from other chapters, opinions vary as to how to best accomplish this goal. Changes may be facilitated through regulatory control, competition in the marketplace, and other factors. Thus, different approaches to managed care have been proposed in the public and private sector. In the process, terms such as effectiveness, evidence-based medicine, and quality have become familiar.

In this chapter, we present a large employer's perspective on the problems of, and some of the popular marketplace strategies for, overseeing managed care, with particular emphasis on common features and differences between regulatory and market forces.

Both the public sector (i.e., government) and the private sector (e.g., the auto industry) play important, often overlapping, roles. Contrary to common perception, the public sector does not equate exclusively with regulation and the private sector does not equate exclusively with market forces. The government, as the largest purchaser in the health industry, plays both regulatory and purchasing roles (see chapters 9 and 12). Similarly, while the private sector behaves primarily as a purchaser, it also acts as a regulator under certain circumstances. In this chapter we explain why we believe market forces are preferable to regulation for managing care. We also explore the expansion of public-private sector partnerships to achieve mutually desired goals, focusing on issues of speed and efficiency, evidence-based decisions, and effectiveness.

Health Care at General Motors

General Motors is the largest private-sector health-care purchaser in the United States, providing coverage to over 1.5 million employees, retirees, and dependents in all fifty states and the District of Columbia. Health-care costs at GM far exceed the amount spent on steel for its vehicles. In 1998, GM's cash expenditures for health care in the United States totaled $3.7 billion. Total booked expenditures were $4.5 billion, including the accounting for post-retiree benefits other than pension (i.e., the SFAS-106 accrual for future retiree costs). Such purchasing power and responsibility for providing coverage to large numbers of individuals afford significant leverage in the health-care industry.

Benefit Options

Approximately 60 percent of GM enrollees choose conventional fee-for-service or indemnity plans, while the remaining 40 percent choose network plans, including PPOs and HMOs. In addition, individuals eligible for coverage may elect no coverage at all. The scope of benefits in GM's U.S. operations is substantial, with an annual total of 31 million health-care transactions. Enrollees receive services that are arranged or provided by 126 HMOs, 80 non-HMO carriers, 6,000 hospitals, 35,000 pharmacies, and 500,000 physicians.[2] In this competitive environment, a range of providers is available to cover the full spectrum of health-care services, from wellness to incipient illness to chronic illness to terminal care.

GM's strategy is to create an environment that rewards consumers, providers, and payers for improved quality and outcomes of care, higher productivity, and lower costs. For most employers, premiums to finance this care are paid by the employees through payroll deductions, while the remaining 80 percent or more is paid ostensibly by the employer.[3] At GM, the employer pays most of the premium for salaried employees and the entire cost for unionized hourly employees. Temporary and contractual employees do not receive health benefits.

Strategies in Managed Care

As a purchaser, GM seeks to provide uniform, high-quality health care while procuring the best value for each dollar spent—a strategy based on value purchasing, partnering, and broad-based coalitions. Similar to existing processes in the automotive industry, managed care at GM rests on the theory that patient-focused care requires the application of best practices and continuous process improvement. "Driving the good" is the goal. This means purchasing the most appropriate care to help patients manage disease, while remaining cognizant of the dynamic nature of medical science. As GM discovered in manufacturing, high costs are often a symptom of poor quality, while improving quality often lowers costs. In the same way, the company contends that higher quality health care should also lead to lower overall costs.

High-Value Paradigm in Health Care

Given the extent of coverage and the diversity in benefits, GM is driven to assure that managed-care providers meet quality and efficiency standards in health-care delivery. General Motors is actively involved with the National Committee for Quality Assurance (see chapter 10), the Foundation for Accountability (FACCT), and the National Forum for Quality Measurement and Reporting, all of which are leaders in the development and reporting of health-care quality measures. Members and participants include representatives of business; government agencies such as the Health Care Financing Administration, the Office of Personnel Management (OPM), the Centers for Disease Control and Prevention (CDC), the Department of Defense, and the Agency for Health Care Policy and Research (AHCPR); and consumer advocates, including the American Association of Retired Persons (AARP) and the AFL-CIO. This collaboration of government, industry, and consumers is an example of the broad-based concern for quality in our nation's health-care system.

Challenges from a Purchaser's Perspective

From a purchaser's perspective, achieving the goals of managed care presents a unique set of challenges. General Motors and all employers that provide health insurance face several important tasks related to purchasing: analyzing alternative health-care services, determining health plan options, defining eligible participants, choosing risk-bearing/funding mechanisms, and complying with statutes, such as ERISA, and coverage continuation requirements included in the Consolidated Omnibus Budget Reconciliation Act of 1985 (COBRA). As a large purchaser, GM also has a civic responsibility to advocate for needed health policy change at the state or national level.[4]

Recognizing the increasing complexity in health care, GM's senior management established a Health Care Initiatives Team in 1994. This team was designed to formulate a strategy to address health-care issues at General Motors and to work with communities to assess health-care quality and cost-effectiveness.

Early studies identified four factors that affect health-care quality and cost: (1) benefit design, (2) government regulations, (3) member behavior and health status, and (4) health-care delivery systems (figure 1). These quality and cost drivers must be addressed in partnership because no single entity has sole control over any of them. General Motors endorses a collaborative approach—involving business, unions, providers, public representatives, government agencies, and consumer advocates—as the most effective route to real and sustainable improvement, not just for GM but for the entire community.

The community approach is increasingly important. At GM, community health reform projects have begun a thorough assessment of and intervention with local health-care delivery systems in five geographic areas: Flint, Michigan; Anderson, Indiana; northeastern Ohio; Dayton, Ohio; and southeastern Michigan. These communities have large numbers of GM employees and some of the highest per-capita health-care costs among GM locations. General

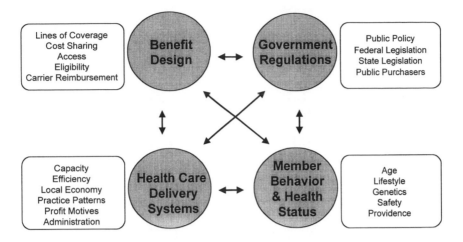

Fig. I. Health-care quality and cost drivers

Motors is working in partnership with its unions, the United Automobile Workers (UAW) and International Union of Electrical Workers (IUE), in this endeavor with formal joint partnerships in Flint, Anderson and northeastern Ohio. In Flint and Anderson, several governmental agencies, including HCFA, have joined the process. This type of partnership is expected to occur in northeastern Ohio as well. Working with health-care experts, the coalitions have completed assessments and have formulated action plans to improve health-care quality and, thereby, reduce costs. The goal is to stimulate the system to improve by creating more awareness of marketplace performance measures among consumers, purchasers, and providers of care. Early evidence shows improvement in both quality and cost in these communities, as reflected in HEDIS data at the community level, satisfaction, and reduction in variability and cost.

Forces of Regulation and Marketplace Competition

Regulatory initiatives and market forces exert tremendous influence on the system of managed care and in defining best practices. In this milieu, the debate continues regarding what approach is best suited to ensure high quality and low cost, as many question the "let the markets rule" philosophy.[5] Although both regulation and competition in the marketplace provide an impetus for lowering costs, the United States still has higher expenses per capita for health care than other countries in the world, with, paradoxically, no evidence of correspondingly superior health outcomes. Legislators have attempted to structure the health-care delivery system with little success. Only recently have purchasers of managed-care products taken the initiative to design a quality paradigm for both managed and fee-for-service health care.[6]

As the largest purchaser in the United States, the government plays a pivotal role in health care. The federal government funds the Medicare program and provides funds to the states for the Medicaid program. Both the federal and state governments provide health-care coverage to their employees.[7] The federal government also pays for health care for those in active military service and their dependents, as well as for many retired and former military personnel.[8] In our view, with its purchasing power, the government can more effectively influence the health-care system through its role as purchaser rather than as regulator. Government regulation suffers from a slow pace and from the influence of political ideologies and special interest groups. As a result, many regulatory initiatives are not based on current, reliable evidence.

From the purchaser's perspective, a paradigm shift needs to occur in the health industry, similar to the one that resulted in a turnaround in the U.S. auto industry. In the past, the auto industry regulated suppliers with specifications for contract delivery. When suppliers were unable to meet industry targets, they were punished by sanctions. The failure of this method of supplier oversight to meet auto industry demands led to a more facilitative relationship with suppliers. Supplier development—actively working with suppliers to understand and meet industry targets—has greatly enhanced quality in the auto industry.

Consistent with GM's philosophy that cost improvement results from quality improvement, GM's programs have focused on improving quality in health care through the purchaser-supplier relationship rather than through sanctions imposed by contract or regulation. At present, GM has a number of initiatives for quality improvement, including the automotive-based program PICOS (Spanish for "mountain peaks"), which aims to help suppliers meet purchaser goals through process improvement. The goal is to work with suppliers to enhance future performance rather than to chasten poor performance. As part of the process, GM collaborates with the Institute for Health Care Improvement to provide access to experts on quality improvement measures. General Motors has contracts with a consulting subsidiary of Kaiser Permanente to provide a team of Kaiser resources to assist in quality improvement and managed-care strategies. The GM/Kaiser Permanente Management Team assesses areas for improvement and provides expertise and access to best-practice resources. Partnerships also exist with benchmark HMOs, plans that meet strict standards for quality and efficiency. GM also has developed partnerships that target specific health-care issues, such as the Enrollment Improvement Process Collaboration with its key HMOs and the Antibiotic Drug Resistance Project with physicians, hospitals, key leaders from medical schools, the

Department of Health, consumer groups, and payers in Michigan and other states. The purchaser works to improve the performance of suppliers and communities, which, in turn, improves the performance of managed care. Thus, through the actions of purchasers, market forces can shape the structure of the health industry with the goal of improving quality of care.

In Defense of Market Forces in Managed Care

From GM's perspective as a purchaser, market forces provide a better alternative to marketplace regulation for three reasons. First, market forces are a faster and more efficient instrument for policy implementation. Second, market forces provide the opportunity for more evidence-based decisions. And finally, market forces are effective.

Market forces are more flexible and adaptable to performance measures, which can quickly change. Market forces may be better suited to drive evidence-based policy into place. They are relatively free of special interest groups and the political machinations that occupy Congress and state regulators and that can influence legislation. Finally, because of the agility associated with the market, particularly in comparison to regulatory efforts, market forces are more effective in addressing health-care issues. The following sections address various types of regulation in relation to market forces and legislation, from the perspective of a purchaser.

Regulation of Benefits

The regulation of benefit design should be driven by efficiency, science, and cost-effectiveness to meet specific and diverse population needs. Allowing the government to determine benefits is bad policy, since its determination may be influenced more by political forces than by scientific evidence. This is the case, for example, when we consider mandated benefit levels for specific diseases or conditions such as mental health, chiropractic, and alternative medicine. Such laws are slow to respond to advances in scientific treatment. Purchasers do not favor government regulation establishing a uniform benefit package since different benefit designs are required to meet the needs of different populations. Benefit design should be based on science and the best allocation of scarce resources. The prudent approach is to foster purchaser efforts to structure a comprehensive benefit plan to meet the needs of its beneficiaries.

Legislated health-care process rules, such as mandates for minimum hospital stays for maternity or mastectomy, cannot effectively regulate appropriate care in a timely manner. The fast pace of change in science and technology demands a more responsive answer than regulation, which can take years to develop and implement. Regulation can be influenced by special interests and may be outdated by the time it is implemented. Reliance on market forces provides health-care suppliers the opportunity to respond rapidly to advances in science and changes in a population's needs in a cost-effective manner and holds providers accountable for quality performance.

Mental health benefits pose a special challenge to purchasers. Instead of mandates for equal benefits for mental health services (known as mental health parity), purchasers prefer to allow the parties (employers, employees, and unions) to choose the most appropriate level of benefits, based on needs, priorities, and resources. Purchasers believe that mental health requires an integrated management approach to design the benefit to meet the population's needs. Regulation cannot accomplish this; purchasers can.

Government mandates also interfere with collective bargaining and free choice. In complex negotiations, unions must balance many priorities, including wages and programs, besides health care. Federal mandates constrain the scope of collective bargaining. Mandates enacted at the state level are largely ineffective because they are preempted by federal law for all self-insured employers. Unless state mandates regulate the "business of insurance," they are also preempted for insured employer-sponsored plans. Hence, the cost of state mandates is disproportionately borne by small companies and individuals who do not obtain coverage through employer-sponsored plans subject to ERISA.

Finally, regulation or legislation that requires a mandatory point-of-service option conflicts with managed-care concepts. The objective of managed care is to create an environment where the public has reasonable choices and the purchaser is accountable for quality and cost-effectiveness. In settings in which these objectives are already met, requiring point-of-service plans can be counterproductive. It can undermine current strategies by reducing the accountability of a health plan or provider group for the committed population. The mandatory point-of-service option can force health-care delivery organizations into the difficult task of managing out-of-network use, a task for which they have inadequate reserves and expertise. If traditional managed-care plans or integrated delivery systems are forced to take risk for out-of-network use, this may ultimately plunge some of these health-care organizations into bankruptcy.

Regulation Directly Affecting Providers

Regulation directly affecting providers includes so-called any willing provider laws. Such laws require a managed-care organization to contract with any provider who meets the conditions imposed by the MCO and is willing to accept the reimbursement levels. Any willing provider laws undermine an MCO's ability to bargain over provider rates and undercut its ability to manage the quality of care provided by caregivers under contract. A provider has no "right" to contract with an MCO any more than any other business or contractor has a "right" to work. Work agreements should be based on merit, not mandates.

Further, health-care delivery requires systems integration and organization for effective managed care. Without a limit to the number and type of providers in a network, the complexity of the organization attempting to manage care would become unwieldy, with a negative impact on quality. A clear provider structure with well-defined boundaries for health-care delivery enables better systems integration and adherence to guidelines and best practices.

From the perspective of the purchaser, mandating participation of certain professionals (e.g., acupuncturists, chiropractors, or lay midwives) is inappropriate, as is mandating coverage for these professionals' services. The objective is to administer high-quality, cost-effective care, not to mandate who renders it. For instance, in some states, chiropractors have lobbied legislators to ensure that the chiropractic profession is represented in MCOs, even in the role of primary care providers. Such legislation is actually provider protection, not consumer protection. If good information on performance is provided to consumers, the market can empower them to select the best care available.

A similar legislature proposal includes nondiscrimination clauses for providers by school of practice, requiring MCOs that cover a certain treatment, test, or procedure to remit payment to any contracted provider who is licensed to render that treatment. However, being licensed to render treatment does not assure quality or cost-effectiveness. Private credentialing and competency requirements of health plans are the most effective means to ensure safe and appropriate care.

Other legislation attempts to address problems that are not real. For example, some legislation dictates requirements for terms that must, and must not, appear in contracts between providers and MCOs. One ostensible purpose of some of this legislation is to avoid gag clauses, which allegedly restrict providers' freedom to discuss with their patients certain issues within the managed-care plan. Organized medicine accused MCOs of forbidding physicians from discussing treatment options with their patients. A General Accounting Office review, however, revealed that gag clauses affecting discussions about treatment are a "red herring" and are virtually nonexistent in actual contracts. Actual clauses are standard antidisparagement or proprietary information clauses common in commercial contracts. Gag clauses are simply a political issue with no practical consequence, except increased costs associated with legal compliance.

Some legislation would require contracting with "essential community providers" such as medical schools or institutions that provide substantial amounts of care to the medically indigent. From the purchaser's perspective, if such providers serve the public good, then financing should come from public funds. In the global economy, a private-sector company cannot stay competitive and afford to contract with providers if that entails paying a premium for their societal missions. However, purchasers do have the responsibility to participate in public policy debates and to work to solve the financing dilemma.

Regulation of Finances

Certain measures to regulate financial matters, including insurer insolvency requirements, are warranted to protect consumers and purchasers. This includes regulating providers who are responsible for health-care costs for care that they do not provide or control. There is a role for appropriate regulation to ensure solvency and compliance with state insurance law. State insurance commissions should regulate insurers and providers, as needed, to protect consumers. In this situation, state regulation of the "business of insurance" needs to be carefully crafted to address true insurance risk, not simply to regulate the fixed payments to the MCO for services that the MCO itself provides. This clarification would ensure that insurance regulations do not expand beyond their appropriate scope.

Risk sharing (also called risk shifting) is an arrangement between MCOs and contracted providers, including physicians, physician organizations, and integrated delivery systems. The attributes of specific risk-sharing models (capitation, subcapitation, incentive payments, and withholds) are best understood and applied in the purchasing negotiation process. With regard to finances, the ultimate regulatory role of government is to protect the consumer from the consequences of insolvency, not to interfere in the negotiation of contracts.

Regulation of Managed-Care Organization Processes and Procedures

Like most regulation in the health industry, the regulation of MCO processes and procedures should be based on speed and efficiency, evidence-based policy, and effectiveness. There is a danger in trying to legislate quality improvement programs. Purchasers can and do require that such programs exist and can influence the content of the program or program processes based on science, customer needs, and practicality. Purchasers can encourage employees to select plans that excel in these features or to drop plans that do not. The problem with legislative mandates is that they can be taken to extremes and can be rigid. Once encoded in law, they can become grounds for litigation. For example, use of clinical guidelines would require use of the latest research-based protocols. At GM, use of such guidelines is specified in an HMO Performance Expectations document. These guidelines vary, depending on local needs and circumstances. This type of flexibility is impossible under set regulations since quality improvement measures are in a state of rapid development. Particularly at this stage in the development of quality measures, market forces can better reward and sanction health plans based on evolving quality improvement performance.

GM agrees that well-structured utilization management or review programs are beneficial. Such programs include mandating that certain processes or standards be used or not used, monitoring underutilization, and promoting the involvement of physicians in the review process. Also, grievance procedures, including time frames, are needed for enrollees or providers who disagree with a payment decision. All of these requirements can be set and monitored by purchasers without regulatory action.

Likewise, due process is desired for providers denied participation in or terminated from an MCO network, along with disclosure of physician selection criteria. However, this process should be no more extensive than any other employment- or contract-related agreement in non-health-care areas of the market. This process can only be implemented in a purchasing environment that satisfies the needs for speed and efficiency, science, and effectiveness.

In consideration of the consumer, GM has incorporated many of the features of the original Consumer Bill of Rights and Responsibilities[9] into its health policy. The president's bill was developed through the consensus of some of the best experts in the country, representing broad constituencies in a nonpolitical process. This deliberative process contrasts with numerous bills in Congress that are driven by political and special interest groups with very little understanding of the potential (negative) impact of many of the provisions. These consumer protections should be incorporated into policy through purchasers, not through regulation. Private purchasers can set specifications, and can be faster and more flexible than legislation, as GM demonstrated in implementing the content of the Consumer Bill of Rights and Responsibilities into its managed-care plans.

Regulation of Information

The Consumer Bill of Rights and Responsibilities also establishes a framework for the regulation of information. The document requires that MCOs disclose certain matters (e.g., physician financial incentives, procedures for access to specialists, how "experimental" treatments are determined) to enrollees and potential enrollees. GM believes this disclosure should be implemented through purchaser requirements, since many proposed regulatory provisions are impossible to administer in light of issues with practicality and timing. Another concern is that legislation might mandate information in a form that would be very difficult, and in many cases impossible, for the consumer to understand. A case in point is the Summary Plan Descriptions required by ERISA, which are difficult for employees to decipher.

Regulations sometimes have unintended consequences. For instance, fear of liability may lead providers or health plans to make poor decisions. Quality and patient safety problems are most often the result of system failures, not negligent or bad people. The only way to fix system problems is to identify them to individuals who have the ability to correct them. This enables the analysis of root causes and the design and implementation of necessary system and process changes. Fear of litigation may suppress identification and disclosure of problems, thus perpetuating potentially dangerous practices. GM is in favor of disclosure of meaningful and understandable information that meets consumer needs in a nonpunitive environment.

The same logic applies to proposed rules requiring that MCOs disclose certain information to the general public upon request (e.g., HEDIS reports and physician or hospital profiles for quality, cost, and utilization data) and requiring that certain information be supplied to state regulators. Specifying content and/or form of disclosures for consistency is reasonable. In fact, much work is being done in the marketplace, through collaboration with the public and private sector, to provide this information in a manner that is credible, timely, and intelligible to the consumer. This is a fluid process, requiring much time and expertise. In terms of development, state-of-the-art outcome measures are only in their infancy. Process measures are further along and rapidly evolving. However, the world of measurement is in a state of tremendous flux, and it is not possible to set regulatory requirements at this point. Mandates would impede, if not halt, progress.

Managed-Care Organization Accountability

Accountability is the underpinning of managed care, addressing responsibility for performance. The need for accountability in managed care makes it essential that consistent, reliable data are available. Accountability results from a market where purchasers and consumers can measure performance and can reward or sanction health plans through public image, market share, and financial incentives. Publicly available provider-specific data should be available, and already are, in performance reports. At the extreme, legal accountability already exists for practices involving fraud or abuse, through the criminal justice system. The complex issue of tort liability is covered in chapter 13.

Mandating Performance Measurement

An important method of assessing managed care is the use of performance measurement; however, these measures change quickly. A distinct advantage of influencing health care via market forces, in contrast to the legislative process, is the flexibility and speed with which the market can respond to issues of performance using state-of-the-art measurement techniques. Measurement is important as it builds evidence for positive change.[10]

GM's strategy for health-care performance measurement focuses on six components: (1) functional outcomes, (2) clinical measures, (3) benefit level,

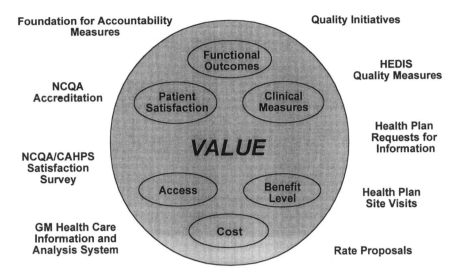

Fig. 2. Health plan value measurement

(4) cost, (5) access, and (6) patient satisfaction (figure 2). Each health plan is scored on each of these six components, and the scores are combined to arrive at a single rating for each plan. In calculating GM's health plan's rating, the quality items (operations review, HEDIS measures, satisfaction survey, and NCQA accreditation) are equally weighted with cost-effectiveness. The health plan ratings form the foundation of GM's communications with its employees and retirees. As noted later, ratings are also used in determining which plans are offered and the level of GM's contributions for salaried employees and retirees.

GM provides a strong financial incentive for salaried employees to select the health plans that perform best on quality. This is a major departure from the traditional flat premium subsidy-based approach used by most purchasers. An array of methods is used to implement the high-quality theme, from financial incentives, plan selection, report cards, and tiered pricing to publicly displayed material encouraging providers to "Be the Best." The goal is to motivate providers toward best practices and continuous improvement and to motivate purchasers toward best quality providers. The salaried HMO migration provides evidence that this quality promotion strategy is working, as illustrated in figure 3. Increased enrollment in "benchmark" and "strong" HMOs and migration out of poor plans show the success of incentives and market forces to influence members toward the top-performing plans. This focus on value from a consumer's point of view is a major improvement in managed care.

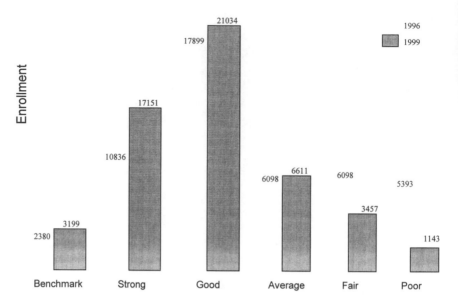

Fig. 3. Salaried HMO migration, in number of enrollees

Continuous Process Improvement

From a purchaser's point of view, continuous process improvement is difficult, if not impossible, to regulate. It has, however, been developed in several managed-care systems, in collaboration between providers and GM in a form of supplier development. As noted earlier, GM uses the PICOS program as one approach to continuous process improvement. PICOS is a collaborative, highly process-oriented improvement model, focusing on three peaks: quality, service, and price. This "workshop" model has been used successfully, including in numerous hospital emergency departments in which teams have reported that as much as 40 percent of operations costs have been removed with rapid improvement in patient flow, improvement in quality, and significantly higher patient satisfaction.

Public-Private Sector Partnering in the Marketplace

The success of managed care hinges on the ability of multiple constituents to work together for the common good. The public and private sectors must work together to promote quality management, share best practices, adopt common performance measures, incorporate value purchasing, and develop new tools.

Cooperative behaviors, rather than punitive measures or regulations, create the optimal environment for consumers, payers, and providers.

An excellent example of this cooperation is the Planning Committee for the Forum for Health Care Quality Measurement and Reporting, which strives to reduce underlying causes of illness, injury, and disability; to research new treatment; to ensure appropriate use of health-care services; to reduce health care errors; to address the undersupply and oversupply of health-care resources; and to increase patients' participation in care. This public-private coalition includes representatives from AARP, the AFL-CIO, AHCPR, Eastman Kodak, GM, HCFA, Henry Ford Health System, the Kaiser Foundation, the National Partnership for Women and Families, the Office of Personnel Management, the U.S. Department of Labor, and Xerox Corporation, among others, all of whom are dedicated to the forum's goals of ensuring the capacity to evaluate and report on quality by promoting consistent data collection; enhancing consumer information and choice about quality; and enabling providers to use data to improve performance. Member organizations agree that consistent data allow meaningful comparisons of providers and plans, which then promotes competition and collaboration on quality. With such public-private sector partnerships, the purchasers, consumers, providers, and researchers help improve managed care much more effectively than could be accomplished by a regulatory scheme.

Conclusion

As the largest nongovernment purchaser of health care in the United States, General Motors has a decided interest in the appropriate management of health care. One strategy is to translate success in the automotive industry to the health industry: to improve quality with subsequent reduction in costs through continuous process improvement. As has been discovered in the auto industry, when purchasers behave as regulators they fail; when they work collaboratively with suppliers they succeed.

Purchasers need to be thoughtful, hardworking drivers of quality principles, or else legislators will fill that void. The purchasing community needs to become more sophisticated and value driven. As the largest purchaser of health care, and as an alternative to its role as regulator, the government can more effectively align with industry as a purchaser. In line with the dynamic nature of health care, only the minimum necessary legislation should be enacted and all legislation should be thoughtfully designed to be amenable to change, as performance, science, and/or technology dictates.

Competitive market forces are preferable to mandated regulation in achieving the goals of managed care for three reasons: (1) speed and efficiency, (2) the opportunity for more evidence-based policy, and (3) effectiveness.

Market force oversight provides more choices to enrollees and allows purchasers to optimize health care. Public-private sector partnerships can facilitate the shift toward supplier development in the market to improve health-care delivery and, ultimately, to improve the health status and behavior of customers.

NOTES

1. M. R. Chassin, "Improving the Quality of Care," *New Eng. J. Med.* 335 (1996): 1060–63.

2. General Motors Corporation, "GM Health Care Fact Sheet," December 1998 and February 9, 1999.

3. J. K. Iglehart, "The American Health Care System—Expenditures," *New Eng. J. Med.* 340 (1999): 70–76. The employee may, in fact, be paying indirectly for the remainder of the premiums, or a portion thereof, through lower wages.

4. J. B. Field and H. T. Shapiro, eds. *Employment and Health Benefits: A Connection at Risk,* U.S. Institute of Medicine, Committee on Employer-Based Health Benefits (Washington, D.C.: National Academy Press, 1993), 123, 147.

5. J. P. Kassirer, "Managed Care and the Morality of the Marketplace," *New Eng. J. Med.* 333 (1995): 50–52.

6. T. Bodenheimer, "The American Health Care System—The Movement for Improved Quality in Health Care," *New Eng. J. Med.* 340 (1999): 488–92.

7. The federal government provides coverage for its employees and their dependents through the Federal Employees Health Benefits Program, a functioning model of wide choice with a defined contribution from the funder. This model is under consideration for the Medicare program.

8. This health care is paid through the Department of Defense, the TRICARE military health system, and Veterans Administration health programs.

9. "Quality First: Better Health Care for All Americans, Appendix A. Consumer Bill of Rights and Responsibilities," Final Report to the President of the United States, U.S. Advisory Commission on Consumer Protection and Quality in the Health Care Industry (Washington, D.C.: U.S. Government Printing Office, 1997).

10. E. C. Nelson, M. E. Splaine, P. B. Batalden, and S. K. Plume, "Building Measurement and Data Collection into Medical Practice," *Ann. Intern. Med.* 128, no. 6 (1998): 460–66.

CHAPTER 9

Medicaid: The Prudent Purchaser

Bruce Bullen

In health care, the prudent purchaser is not just the consumer. The prudent purchaser must also be the organization (employer or government agency) that makes buying decisions on behalf of the consumer—whether the consumer is an employee or beneficiary. The purchaser's objective should be to obtain value. The best value is the best combination of quality and cost. In order to obtain health-care value, the prudent purchaser must define quality, measure it, seek to improve it, and exert market leadership.

A basic premise of this approach is that prudent purchasing of health care means purchasing managed care. Purchasing *un*managed care is not prudent. It costs too much, and its quality is suspect. Who does the managing, toward what end, how, and how tightly? These are all questions that can be debated. What is beyond debate is that prudent purchasing of managed care is the best way—the *only* way—to obtain value in today's health-care world, and probably tomorrow's world as well.

To obtain value, quality must be defined. For the prudent purchaser of health care, defining quality is no easy task. For example, what is quality in mental health care? The number of providers? Their credentials? Is it the number of visits provided? The percentage of enrollees receiving mental health services? The degree of consumer satisfaction with the care received? The number of patients who report improvement in their ability to cope with the stress of daily life? The specifics of what constitutes quality may vary from purchaser to purchaser. What does not vary is the necessity to make the determination.

Every important element of what the purchaser thinks quality is must be defined. This can be an arduous process. It requires listening to consumers—really listening. It requires consultation with health plans and providers. It requires a high degree of collaboration. And, at its heart, it requires pushing the health-care system down paths it is reluctant to travel.

Once quality is defined, the prudent purchaser seeking to obtain quality must express those definitions in purchasing specifications. These specifications spell out for potential vendors the purchaser's expectations. My agency's health plan purchasing specifications, for instance, contain hundreds of pages. They cover structure, process, and outcomes. They include access, network management, clinical and quality management, reporting, financial stability, and financial management—all the elements of quality as we see it.

An important aspect of defining quality is deciding how to measure it. Measurement is the key to prudent purchasing. Without it, there is no way to determine whether quality was obtained and no way of managing toward higher quality. The measures we use today in health care are rudimentary. The challenge of prudent purchasing is to push the entire world of health care in the direction of developing meaningful measures of quality. Part of that challenge is that there are still those (usually providers) who insist that health-care quality cannot be measured, although they claim to "know it when they see it."

As for the rest of us, as prudent purchasers we must, for now, rely on the measurements that are currently available to us: HEDIS and other data, satisfaction surveys, and so on. They are a beginning, but better measures, those that are more outcome oriented, are needed. Prudent purchasers must keep up the pressure that will lead to the development and use of such measures.

Health-care quality can be improved. The health-care system is not a black box; it can be made to improve through targeted, practical interventions. Quality improvement is a process, and it must be managed. This is another reason why the prudent purchaser looks toward managed care.

There is, however, no easy way to obtain better quality. Quality improvements are hard-won and require realism, cooperation, and accountability on the part of purchasers, plans, and providers. Improvement takes time, and the only way to know whether you have succeeded is to identify opportunities for improvement, set measurable goals, and measure—and remeasure—performance. Unfortunately, this means that the process is often prosaic and the improvements incremental. But the results are worth it.

Here are some examples from our experience in Massachusetts:

- During a two-year period, the number of complex births for members in our HMO program fell from 5.6 per 1,000 female members to 3.19 per 1,000.
- One of our HMOs reduced the rate of premature births from 19 percent to 2.3 percent.
- Another HMO developed a program targeting children with asthma. Both inpatient admissions and emergency room visits were reduced by 50 percent.
- Our primary care case-management program reduced asthma-related hospital admissions by 38 percent.
- The behavioral health penetration rate (that is, the percentage of enrollees receiving some care) increased 20 percent among HMO members as a result of our making this a focus of quality improvement efforts.

- Our managed behavioral health program increased access to community-based services in lieu of hospitalization. For adults in an intensive clinical management program, days in the community increased from 254 per year to 329. For children, the increase was from 259 days to 338 days.
- Hospital readmission rates within thirty days for members with mental illness decreased from 14 percent to 7 percent.

At the same time, we achieved high satisfaction rates among enrollees in managed-care plans:

- Ninety-five percent of parents reported satisfaction with the ease of scheduling a doctor visit when their child was sick.
- Ninety-seven percent gave favorable ratings to the quality of care given to their children.
- Ninety-two percent gave favorable ratings regarding the quality of their own care.

And our enrollees are getting the care they need:

- Eighty-eight percent of children up to age nineteen had at least one primary care visit in the last year.
- Seventy-eight percent of children between the ages of three and six had a well-child visit in the last year.
- Ninety percent of pregnant women enrolling in HMOs had their first prenatal visit within six weeks of enrollment.
- Eighty-eight percent of pregnant women in HMOs had their first prenatal visit during the first trimester of their pregnancy.

The prudent purchaser must put in place the elements of a good quality management system: negotiated performance goals, member satisfaction surveys and focus groups, independent external reviews, continuous quality improvement systems, data reporting, and consequences for underachievers. Then the prudent purchaser must use these elements effectively, keeping in mind that the system should not be micromanaged or made to respond to unrealistic expectations.

State Medicaid programs provide some of the best examples of the kinds of quality improvement made possible under this prudent purchaser model. Most Medicaid programs are in the process of transforming themselves from passive, regulated bill payers to active, flexible purchasers of the kind of health care that meets the needs of Medicaid consumers. As more Medicaid programs purchase managed systems of care through health plans, long-standing problems are beginning to be solved. Such problems include access to obstetricians or gynecologists for low-income mothers, Early and Periodic Screening, Diagnosis, and Treatment (EPSDT) screening rates for their children, access to culturally competent providers, and the prevalence of untreated asthma among the Medicaid population. Improvements in these areas are being made every year in many states.

State Medicaid programs have pioneered a public-private partnership on managed-care quality. Several states have been employing HEDIS measures for years, and Medicaid participation in the development of HEDIS 3.0 ensured the incorporation into this system of Medicaid-relevant measures. Many states have made substantial investments in consumer satisfaction surveys, and almost all states now monitor disenrollments, manage grievance processes, and employ toll-free number consumer complaint mechanisms. Some states are collaborating with private purchasing groups to obtain additional purchasing leverage. All this is over and above traditional licensing, accreditation, and participation standards.

Medicaid programs are using managed-care organizations as cost-effective tools to improve access and consumer satisfaction for Medicaid enrollees. Through the use of managed-care organizations and principles, real, measurable improvements are being made in many states in the quality of health care for Medicaid recipients. Managed care offers unparalleled promise as a tool for achieving the ultimate goal of the Medicaid program: to mainstream the poor into the private health-care system in a way that meets their needs fully and avoids a two-tier health-care system.

This promise can only be realized if Medicaid programs are free to employ quality improvement strategies as purchasers and to take advantage of market changes. Unrealistic statutory restrictions on the use of managed care will have the unintended effect of diluting these efforts. Attempts to legislate quality or increase consumer protection should recognize the strides that prudent purchasing has made and should protect the ability of purchasers, including Medicaid, to obtain value. And when those attempts are thinly disguised efforts by providers to improve their bargaining position with managed-care organizations, prudent purchasers should be outspoken in identifying whose interests are being served, and whose are not, in particular the needs and interests of consumers.

The most difficult, challenging, exciting, and rewarding part of being a prudent purchaser is exerting leadership. The prudent purchaser is not a passive buyer who merely selects the best value from among the choices offered. The prudent purchaser is one who has a vision of what health care can, and should, be and who works creatively with others to bring that vision to life. The prudent purchaser imagines what health care should look like ten years from now for the people on whose behalf the purchaser acts. That purchaser thinks about access, outcomes, patient dignity, increased self-sufficiency, and greater patient involvement in care decisions. He or she thinks about all the elements of quality that could be improved and about what constitutes a reasonable cost for a system that could provide what is needed. That picture is the purchaser's vision. The challenge now is to make it *real*.

The prudent purchaser drives the marketplace toward objectives that the purchaser sets. The process may take time. It will require allies. It will encounter resistance: resistance from some providers, from some health plans, and from some advocates.

It is therefore necessary to work with other purchasers to achieve one's vision. In Massachusetts, it was the Medicaid agency that provided the leadership that led to the formation of the Massachusetts Healthcare Purchasers Group—an organization that coordinates purchasing strategies on behalf of nearly 2 million of our state's 6 million people. Together, public agencies and private employers are working toward a vision of higher quality, more affordable health care for the people of our state. Interestingly, it is the public purchasers who are the most aggressive in pursuit of that vision. We believe that the efforts of the Purchasers Group will have greater impact on the quality and affordability of health care than will anything else that occurs in our state in the next few years.

My advice to those who would be prudent purchasers is this: Join a purchaser group if one exists in your state. Help make it an effective manager of managed care. If no such group exists, get together with other purchasers and create one. Working together you will have far more strength than you will working separately. Within your purchaser group, take bold positions with a view toward nothing less than revolutionary changes in the delivery of health care. Drive the health-care marketplace toward high performance networks that will improve quality and increase affordability.

Remember, prudent doesn't mean timid.

Editors' Note: The editors posed a few key questions to the author.

In what ways is a state Medicaid program purchasing health care similar to a private employer purchasing health care? In what ways is it different?

BULLEN: While there are many similarities between a state Medicaid program and a large employer that offers health insurance to employees, there are some significant differences as well.

In the process of selecting health plans, Medicaid programs and employers weigh many of the same factors. However, because Medicaid is a government program, the Medicaid process is generally more formal than that used by most private employers. Other functions that are similar include negotiating rates, disseminating information about choices, measuring quality, and resolving member complaints. One major difference is that purchasing health care is our principal purpose. For private employers, it is a "fringe" issue when compared to their principal business purpose.

Other differences include:

- the scale—Massachusetts Medicaid is ten times bigger than the largest employer
- the benefit package—Medicaid is a rich benefit package with no copayments or deductibles, unlimited mental health coverage, and long-term care
- the necessity to include "safety net" providers in the provider network
- federally imposed upper payment limits
- no "work site" communication with enrolled individuals
- lower literacy rates and reading comprehension levels among beneficiaries
- many more non-English speaking people, making communication a challenge
- proportionately more seriously ill and disabled persons
- less assertive population
- operating in the public spotlight (advocates, media, legislature)

Does the state, as a unit of government, have more leverage than a private employer to offer protection to its managed-care enrollees?

BULLEN: The law does provide additional safeguards for Medicaid, and Medicare, beneficiaries. While there are some advantages to being a unit of state government, there are some disadvantages as well. The principal advantages of a Medicaid program have less to do with being part of state government and more to do with size. There is also a special "moral authority" that accrues to the state when it is purchasing on behalf of the neediest segments of society. Whether out of altruism, mission, or fear of bad publicity, many plans and providers respond differently to the state than to private purchasers. Another factor is a generally unfounded concern that to alienate one part of state government is to jeopardize relations with other parts as well.

Many employers offer their employees a choice among a variety of health-care programs. What is your position on states mandating participation in a single managed-care program for their Medicaid beneficiaries (that is, not offering a choice)? Should states offer their Medicaid beneficiaries managed care as one option among a variety of health-care programs?

BULLEN: Our belief is that beneficiaries should have a meaningful choice. Massachusetts contracts with several health plans and operates its own managed-care plan (a primary care case management program) in order to provide such a choice of plans. For most of our population, we do not offer the option of a nonmanaged plan. We believe that offering well-run managed-care plans that operate under our contract management is a better way to provide services than through an unmanaged-care system.

Not all physicians are willing to accept Medicaid patients. Does offering managed care to Medicaid beneficiaries improve or reduce access to physicians for this population? Is there a difference in this effect between urban and rural populations?

BULLEN: Offering managed-care plans increases access because some physicians who do not accept Medicaid patients are part of the provider panels of one or more of our managed-care plans. Beneficiaries therefore have access to a greater number of providers.

CHAPTER 10

NCQA: Using Market Pressure to Promote Quality in Managed Care

Margaret E. O'Kane

Twenty years ago, health maintenance organizations were still more of an idea than an industry. They were isolated efforts to care for Americans by maintaining health through a focus on disease prevention and health promotion. Today, managed care is the norm, with more than 80 million privately insured enrollees in HMOs and tens of millions more enrolled in other managed-care offerings such as point-of-service plans, preferred provider organizations, "managed indemnity" plans, and other products.

The rapid expansion of managed care into the mainstream has created some concern and with it a substantial demand for quality assurance. The concern reflects the realities of managed care: limitations on provider choice, incentives that may limit the delivery of appropriate care, and the introduction of a third party into the doctor-patient relationship. At the same time, few wish to abandon the promise of managed care—to control costs and keep people healthy. In this context, employers and consumers have increasingly demanded that adequate quality assurance mechanisms be established to provide protection against the risks inherent in managed-care systems. The hope, of course, is to realize the promise of managed care without surrendering ourselves to questionable quality. These quality assurance mechanisms are quite diverse, but they can be divided into two general types: regulatory initiatives and attempts to use market forces to encourage the delivery of high-quality care.

Clearly, an effective national approach to quality assurance should take advantage of both regulation and market forces. The danger is that we come to rely exclusively on one or the other. Nevertheless, some recent legislative initiatives would seem to do just that: replace successful private market efforts with new government bureaucracies. The idea of using the regulatory might of the federal government to, in effect, mandate quality into managed care seems appealing in its simplicity—establish the rules and quality will follow. In practice, however, the sought-after improvement proves chimerical. While regulation is an important component of an overall approach to promoting quality improvement, regulation must be coupled with other well-tested, market-based means to the same ends.

The National Committee for Quality Assurance, working with purchasers, consumers, health plans, and others, has successfully worked to leverage market pressure to promote quality in managed care. By any measure, NCQA's impact on the market has been great: important quality improvement and information systems have been built up around NCQA's performance measurement and accreditation programs. Millions of Americans now receive standardized information about how well their health plans perform on key measures of quality. Over half of the nation's HMOs (covering three out of four Americans enrolled in HMOs) have voluntarily submitted to NCQA's rigorous survey process. Finally, demonstrating quality across the industry has become a prerequisite for market success—or even for the opportunity to bid for certain business. And yet NCQA holds no regulatory authority. Our success is instead based on the collective clout of the large employers and public purchasers whose mandates to participate in NCQA's programs send a clear message to health plans: focus on quality or we'll find coverage elsewhere. That message resonates. The good news for health-care purchasers and consumers is that NCQA has been able to use that pressure to effect real change in managed care. Among leading HMOs, the basis for competition is clearly shifting from cost to value and quality. There's still important work to be done, of course. Price remains the main factor in most health-care purchasing decisions. And quality is by no means uniformly high in the industry, as NCQA's 1997 and 1998 *State of Managed Care Quality* reports clearly show. But things are moving in the right direction and at an accelerating pace.

A comprehensive discussion of the appropriate balance between regulation and market-based approaches in promoting quality is beyond the scope of this chapter. Instead I will briefly review some of the limits of regulatory approaches and then look in more detail at how NCQA has marshaled the support, expertise, and purchasing power of employers, consumers, and others to help redefine the environment for managed-care plans so that it rewards excellent care and service. I will also look in detail at NCQA's rigorous accreditation and performance measurement programs, which are the tools most commonly used to evaluate the quality and performance of managed systems of care.

Regulatory Approaches: The Limitations

Experience with regulation suggests that it has an important, but *limited*, role in assuring quality in managed care for the following reasons.

1. *Regulation doesn't promote innovation.* The processes of developing, modifying, and implementing regulations can be slow and plagued by

inertia. To this extent, regulations may fail to encourage or even permit creative approaches to quality assessment and oversight and may be slow to recognize innovation when it has occurred. By contrast, existing market approaches already have built-in mechanisms to ensure that new approaches to, or ideas about, quality assessment can be incorporated into oversight programs on a regular basis.

2. *Regulatory processes are essentially political.* Establishing regulations is a political process, subject to the influence of political pressure. As a result, political processes have a tendency to promote the status quo; regulators may be slow to embrace strategies that rock the boat even when change is plainly necessary.

3. *Low regulatory thresholds would offer scant protection and would not encourage quality improvement.* That an independent body can develop and maintain more effective and timely standards and measures than a regulatory body seems obvious. In other industries, states and federal governments have demonstrated a reluctance to intervene at the margins of acceptable performance despite their obligation to protect the public. Where the state's authority rests in its ability to terminate a license and put an organization out of business, the level of evidence required for action may be so high that it is only in the most egregious cases that action is taken. This limits the potential of governmental actors to assure—and certainly to improve—the quality of managed-care plans. Market pressure can effectively encourage improvement not only at the margin but across the whole system and even among high performers.

Are market forces a reliable alternative? Competitive pressure can and should be the primary force driving quality improvement in managed care, as it has been in the markets for other goods and services in the United States. However, there seems little doubt that the market for health-care services is different. Health care is not a commodity of uniform price and quality, and there are many aspects of health-care purchasing that are unique and to which conventional economic theory does not apply. It is appropriate, therefore, to include in our discussion of market mechanisms for quality assurance in managed care a consideration of the two assumptions upon which that discipline depends, namely, (1) that given economic incentives to improve quality, MCOs will attempt to do so, and (2) that given adequate information about the quality and performance of managed-care firms, purchasers and consumers will gravitate toward those organizations that provide the highest quality.

There seems little reason to doubt that managed-care organizations respond to economic incentives in much the same way as do other firms. To this extent, quality is assured if purchasers and consumers are willing to reward higher quality firms with their business (assuming that purchasers and consumers have the ability to recognize those managed-care organizations that are providing higher quality).

Is it true that purchasers and consumers will vote, with their pocketbooks, for higher quality managed-care firms? This issue seems less clear. On the one hand, an increasing number of corporations (e.g., Xerox, Digital, General Motors, Delta Airlines, IBM, Mobil, PepsiCo, and McDonald's) are mandating that managed-care firms interested in their business distinguish themselves by achieving accreditation from an objective evaluator such as NCQA. On the other hand, price was still clearly the more important market force in 1998, copious media coverage of quality issues notwithstanding.

What does this mean? Clearly it means that competition *is* possible in the market for managed-care services. While some have argued that the managed-care market is imperfect (and we have no doubt that it is), it is nevertheless competitive. In fact, it is aggressively price-competitive. But that does not establish that competition based on quality is impossible. First, in the absence of information about quality, it is hard to understand how anyone might expect to see anything *but* price competition. And to a very large extent, consumers and employers are only now learning that quality information is available and about how to use it. More than that, it is difficult to predict what will be the basis for competition when truly competitive prices have been achieved (and managed care becomes something of a commodity). It seems more than likely that in the future only small differences in price will distinguish one managed-care firm from another. When that is so, quality will be the feature that distinguishes one MCO from another in the marketplace.

It also seems likely that growing consumer interest and ongoing consumer education will spark quality-based competition in the near future to a greater extent than it has in the past. As managed care becomes a reality for more consumers, a critical mass will become interested in quality, and it will move to the fore of the MCO agenda. In fact, consumer interest in quality—sparked by the growth of HMOs (especially among the influential elderly, for whom health-care quality is an issue of paramount importance) and fueled by the greater availability of information about quality—may prove to be the force that drives the quality-competitive marketplace.

The NCQA Approach: Accreditation and Performance Measurement

Two efforts under way at NCQA—NCQA accreditation and HEDIS performance measurement—provide information to purchasers and consumers to help inform their health-plan selection decisions. As this information becomes more readily available—and as more potential users realize that it is available—we believe that competition based on quality will become even more evident than it is already. What follows is a brief explanation of each initiative.

Accreditation

NCQA's accreditation program is a strategy for evaluating whether a health plan operates in a manner that is expected to result in care and service that meet the needs of its membership and whether it can demonstrate that it delivers high-quality care and meets certain performance targets. NCQA accreditation is organized around standards (which evaluate systems and processes) and performance measures (which evaluate clinical effectiveness). NCQA's accreditation program focuses on five main areas.

- *Ensuring access and service.* Is the health plan proactive in terms of ensuring that members get the care and service they need? Do members understand their rights and responsibilities and the policies and procedures of the plan? Are there effective complaint and grievance processes? Do they motivate action? Is there closure?
- *Ensuring qualified providers.* Does the health plan rigorously check that providers have the credentials they claim to have? Can the health plan document that appropriate credentials have been verified? Does the health plan incorporate information from ongoing performance reviews of providers into recredentialing decisions?
- *Staying healthy.* Does the plan effectively promote preventive care to maintain the health of its members? Is there evidence that guidelines for preventive care are developed and communicated to providers and patients as appropriate? Is there evidence that the success of preventive care is monitored? Is there evidence of improvement?
- *Getting better.* Does the plan work to help sick or injured members recover as quickly and fully as possible? Is there appropriate follow-up? Are members recovering as would be expected in a well-functioning health plan?
- *Living with illness.* Do people get help for living with ongoing illness? What measures does the health plan take to protect sick members' quality of life? How well does it monitor members' functional status? Are appropriate mental or behavioral health supports available?

In addition to being evaluated in these five areas, plans are also required to submit performance data for several HEDIS measures (see the following section for more information about HEDIS). NCQA uses these data to determine whether health plans are achieving important care and service objectives. Compliance with standards and a plan's HEDIS data factor into NCQA's ultimate accreditation decision, and summary information from both parts of the survey is made available to employers and consumers. This two-part survey of each plan yields a complete, objective picture of plan quality.

The accreditation process involves a site review, undertaken by a team of physician and nonphysician quality experts. Typically, three to five reviewers work on the process for three or more days. Data from the on-site review are summarized in a report, which is reviewed by a committee of senior physicians and executives from the industry. This committee then makes the accreditation determination and assigns the plan one of five different status levels—excellent, commendable, accredited, provisional, and denial. The standards are high, deliberately so. Accreditation is a rigorous process, and a health plan truly must be capable of operating at a high level across all critical functions in order to achieve an excellent or commendable designation.

HEDIS

Before HEDIS measures were incorporated into NCQA's accreditation program with the release of the 1999 MCO Accreditation Standards, the two programs grew up separately, with accreditation focusing on a review of systems and processes and HEDIS looking at performance—two sides of the same coin. HEDIS, in contrast to NCQA accreditation, is a set of standardized performance measures designed to ensure that purchasers and consumers have the information they need to reliably compare the performance of managed health plans on an "apples-to-apples" basis.

HEDIS is based on the idea of standardization. There are dozens of different ways health plans might measure immunization rates, mammography rates, member satisfaction, smoking cessation, utilization, access, and so on. The rigorously defined technical specifications in HEDIS, however, help ensure that health plans across the country all calculate these measures in the same way. HEDIS defines not only how to calculate each measure but how and when to generate the sample on which it is based and the process by which independent auditors must review each data element for accuracy. About 90 percent of the nation's health plans report at least some HEDIS data.

NCQA's long-term vision for performance measurement is one in which the full range of information about health-plan performance is available to allow purchasers and consumers to make comparisons and to support health-plan efforts to improve. To achieve that vision, we have focused our efforts in five areas.

- *Technical specifications.* HEDIS is a precisely specified information set that serves as the industry's standard tool for performance evaluation. It is responsive to the needs of purchasers, consumers, and health plans.
- *The audit process.* NCQA's HEDIS Compliance Audit program assures that production of HEDIS data conforms with the precise specifications laid

out by NCQA and that HEDIS data are credible to purchasers and consumers. As HEDIS data become more available, it will be critical to assure that results do not misrepresent performance and thereby lead users to incorrect conclusions.

- *NCQA's Quality Compass.*™ NCQA's database of HEDIS and accreditation information brings data from hundreds of plans together, to make data more accessible to users and to permit benchmarking and analysis.
- *Consumer research.* NCQA investigates the information needs of consumers to assure that future generations of HEDIS will be responsive and targeted.
- *Data distribution.* NCQA is exploring ways to make HEDIS data more meaningful and accessible to users.

HEDIS 1999 includes about fifty-five measures that focus on a broad array of issues ranging from clinical process to financial performance. About 90 percent of HMOs will report the range of measures—as part of NCQA's accreditation program—internally for quality improvement purposes or to employers and NCQA's Quality Compass. HEDIS covers a broad range of issues that matter not only to private purchasers but also to those who manage the Medicare and Medicaid programs and to those who receive care regardless of whether they are privately or publicly insured. As such, HEDIS data underlie almost all health-plan report cards appearing in local newspapers, employer-distributed benefits material, or health-plan marketing material. HEDIS 1999 is far more outcome-oriented than were any of its earlier versions. The set of measures is organized into eight "domains," areas on which purchasers, consumers, policymakers, and others have told us that measures need to focus.

- *Effectiveness of care.* Is the care provided achieving the results we expect it to achieve?
- *Accessibility and availability of care.* Is care available to those who need it, without inappropriate barriers and delay?
- *Satisfaction with the experience of care.* Is the experience of care satisfying as well as clinically effective?
- *Cost of care.* Is the care of "high value"?
- *Stability of the health plan.* Is the health plan stable? Or will members experience the sort of change (e.g., provider turnover) that could disrupt care?
- *Informed health-care choices.* Is the health plan successful at helping members to be active and informed partners in health-care decisions?
- *Use of services.* How are resources used? Is there evidence of too much—or too little—care?
- *Plan descriptive information.* How is the plan organized? What types of doctors participate and how many?

The measures in HEDIS are intended to serve as national reporting requirements for managed-care firms. In some sense they already do: nearly three hundred health plans reported data to Quality Compass in 1998. NCQA made much of those data available to the press, who in turn used the data to generate local and national report cards.

As previously noted, HEDIS measures are precisely specified so that rules for calculation are unambiguous. In addition to these "reporting set" measures, there are many additional measures that are included as a "testing set." Measures in the testing set are used for evaluation. They are measures that were felt to be important and promising but for which significant concern existed about their usefulness for health-plan comparison in 1998–99. The objective of the testing set is to create a mechanism to generate evidence about the characteristics of these measures, so as to better evaluate their potential usefulness for future generations of HEDIS and to refine those measures that evidence suggests have great utility. It is also to signal where HEDIS is headed to provide managed-care firms with more lead time to prepare care management and information systems to address areas that are not addressed by the current HEDIS reporting set.

The evolution and development of HEDIS is guided by a broad-based committee—the Committee on Performance Measurement (CPM)—whose members were chosen to reflect the diversity of constituencies that performance measurement must serve: purchasers (both public and private), consumers, organized labor, medical providers, public health officials, and health plans. Other experts also sit on the CPM and bring to it additional expertise in the areas of quality management and performance measurement. Working to forge a consensus among these diverse groups about what can and should be measured ensures that HEDIS reflects the needs of all constituencies.

Driving Markets with Data

This chapter has thus far looked at the programs—accreditation and HEDIS— through which NCQA generates information about health plans. For such programs to function effectively in tandem with regulation, it is important to consider how that information is made available and how it is used. In order to be useful to purchasers and consumers of health care, information has to be presented to them in a way that is comprehensible and has to be available to them when they need it.

Employers

There are countless examples of employers and organizations that have been successful in making quality and performance information available. Several large companies provide highly customized reports to their employees. Some employers' reports go so far as to provide employees with information on the health plans that operate only within the zip codes in which they live. This saves workers from having to wade through a nationwide or regional list of plans, benefit packages, and performance data. In other cases, employers provide electronic access to the information, with leading employers setting up web sites with information about available health plans' NCQA accreditation information and HEDIS data.

Coalitions and the Media

Performance information has been released as HEDIS report cards by purchasing coalitions and by the lay press. We have watched, and participated, as coalitions of purchasers and health plans—such as the California Cooperative HEDIS Reporting Initiative (CCHRI) and the New England HEDIS Coalition—have produced HEDIS report cards and as large and influential employers have made data on plans available to employees at open enrollment. HEDIS and NCQA accreditation results have been published in specialized publications (e.g., *Health Pages*, a journal providing health-care and health plan information for consumers) and even in the lay press (e.g., *Barron's*, *USA Today*, and *U.S. News and World Report*). Accreditation data are also available from NCQA; more than thirty thousand organizations and individuals seek that information monthly.

Quality Compass

Efforts to make information even more widely available are under way. In August 1996, NCQA offered the first Quality Compass, a national database of NCQA accreditation and HEDIS data from many of the nation's health plans (about three hundred plans participated in Quality Compass in 1998). Quality Compass is designed to be user-friendly and permits easy comparison of one plan to another or to national or regional benchmarks. The CD-ROM format permits users to sort and print data in a variety of ways. Employers, consultants, health plans, and particularly the media have all found Quality Compass to be an invaluable resource for comparing health plans.

State Report Cards

Finally, a small number of states release performance information for public use. New Jersey and Maryland both released health plan performance data in a consumer-friendly report card format in 1998, and many other states are engaged in similar efforts. Clearly the state can be a powerful force for moving information to the public, and some states have already begun to provide leadership in this regard. Notably, five states, Alabama, Iowa, New York, Ohio, and Tennessee, also require NCQA accreditation of plans serving state employees, an essentially cost-free means of leveraging the massive purchasing power of the state to promote quality in managed health care.

For the purposes of our original question—how we should balance regulatory versus market approaches in promoting quality in managed care—these examples are significant. In each case, the motivation and the result are clear. The effective distribution of information about health plan quality can exert, and *is* exerting, market pressure to promote quality. And it seems unlikely that at this point this positive trend will reverse. By actively seeking and using NCQA-supplied data, consumers and employers are delivering an unambiguous message to the managed-care community: quality matters.

What Does the Future Hold?

What has been, and what will be, the impact of the release of more information to the public? We offer the following short list.

1. *Health plans will feel increasing pressure to demonstrate excellence and to improve the quality of care and service that they provide.* Increasing this pressure is, of course, the primary objective of producing and releasing quality information. We see this trend already and expect to see it grow over time, as more information becomes available and as more of those for whom it is intended recognize that it is available and become familiar with its use.

2. *Other health-care organizations will feel the same pressure that health plans do.* To some extent, this is a consequence of parallel efforts to measure and report on the performance of hospitals, physicians, and other components of the health-care system. Some of these efforts are under way but have not moved as quickly as have those just described. But to some extent, pressure will rise elsewhere within the system, because managed-care firms, which are being held accountable for results, have recognized that they need information about the quality of care and service delivered to their members from those with whom they contract, if they are going to manage quality the way they are now expected to. This "transmitted" pressure is a positive force, one that will help to improve quality at the provider level and to coordinate quality improvement efforts at different levels of the system.

3. *Organizational strategic planning will focus on improving performance in those areas where information is released to the public.* There is both an upside and a downside to this. The visibility of results will lead to the allocation of resources to areas where improvement is evidently most

needed. As a result, health plans and others will invest in improving clinical and service performance. The risk, however, is that investment will be limited to areas where there are performance measures; in other words, *only* what gets measured will get done. As it is impossible to require the public release of information for all issues that might be important, there is some risk that important issues will not get the attention they deserve, because no public reporting is required.

There are strategies for dealing with the possibility that areas lacking published performance measures will be ignored in efforts to improve quality. One, of course, is to assure that expert evaluation of organizations continues to be a component of the overall system for evaluation. To the extent that experts are involved in detailed inspection of a health-care organization, there is an opportunity to assure that the organization's efforts to manage quality are not too narrowly focused. Even so, those who develop strategies for public reporting are well advised to consider the responsibility that that activity implies. Laying out the public reporting agenda is tantamount to setting strategic priorities for health-care organizations, and the potential to do harm by misdirecting resources is real and must be considered.

In the long run, the consumer will become a smarter purchaser; this will move quality assurance deep into the system. While we expect the availability of comparative information to assist consumers in making choices more in line with their preferences—and to see a positive impact on the marketplace as a result—we think the longer-term impact of the public release of information will be even greater. We believe—and our work with consumers suggests that it is more than an article of faith—that performance information can have a powerful effect to stimulate consumers to become more aware of the issues that are important to them. Report cards are a tool both for communicating information and for encouraging consumers to learn about related issues. Knowing about the mammography rates of two plans, for example, tells consumers something about the priorities of those health plans and about their success achieving results in line with their priorities. But information about mammography rates also raises awareness of the importance of mammography and of the health plan's role in assuring that women seek and receive preventive care. This awareness will help consumers ask the questions that matter. Educated consumers will raise levels of accountability to unprecedented heights. Hand in hand with appropriate regulation, market forces have already made real gains in quality across the industry, and more are sure to follow.

NOTE

This paper was written in 1997 and subsequently edited in January 1999.

CHAPTER 11

The American Association of Health Plans: Representing the Industry

American Association of Health Plans

This chapter provides an overview of how two types of health plans—health maintenance organizations and preferred provider organizations—are regulated. It examines a broad range of regulation, including traditional regulation (such as state licensure requirements and Medicare program participation requirements) as well as private accreditation requirements and separate purchaser-imposed requirements. In this context, regulation is defined as rules and requirements that govern health plan behavior.

Sources of Regulation

Health plans are subject to regulation by numerous entities at the federal and state levels as well as by private-sector entities. For example, in addition to the four major federal regulatory agencies–the Department of Health and Human Services (HHS), the Department of Labor (DOL), the Department of Defense (DOD), and the Office of Personnel Management—the Internal Revenue Service, the Department of Justice, and the Federal Trade Commission, to mention a few, also have regulatory responsibilities over health plans. State regulators include insurance and health departments as well as labor and personnel departments. Also, health plans increasingly are meeting standards established by private accrediting organizations as well as specific employer requirements.

Editors' Note: The following chapter was contributed by the Association of American Health Plans, the trade organization that represents managed-care companies in the United States. The chapter describes current government regulation of managed care and reports the results of a cost-of-regulation analysis performed by the Barents Group LLC consulting company that estimates the likely financial impact of various scenarios of managed-care regulation.

Federal Regulation

As mentioned, at least four federal agencies establish rules and requirements that affect health plans. The Department of Health and Human Services, acting primarily through the Health Care Financing Administration, serves as a purchaser of health-care coverage and as a regulator. Under the HMO Act of 1973, HCFA sets standards affecting key aspects of plan design and operations. Designation as a "federally qualified" HMO is voluntary and can be viewed as a federal seal of approval as well as protection from state laws that conflict with requirements of the federal HMO Act.

HCFA also purchases and regulates health-care coverage for Medicare beneficiaries who choose to enroll in health plans. An HMO or, beginning in 1999, PPO that participates in Medicare must be licensed and must meet various layers of requirements in every state in which it seeks to enroll beneficiaries. It also must meet a separate set of federal requirements and standards designed to assure its suitability for the Medicare market. Where there is a direct conflict between a Medicare requirement and state law, the federal rule prevails at least for the Medicare portion of a health plan's operations.

HCFA determines whether a health plan meets program requirements by conducting an initial "desk review" of its application and then verifying information during an on-site visit. Continuing compliance is monitored through follow-up visits at the end of a health plan's first year in the Medicare market and at least every two years thereafter. HCFA review, including on-site review, also is mandated when a plan seeks to expand its service area.

In addition to establishing federal requirements for health plans participating in state Medicaid programs, the federal government also has an oversight role. It reviews contracts between states and health plans and also reviews the written plan submitted to HCFA by the state for assurances that Medicaid managed-care programs and participating plans will meet federal contractual requirements. HCFA investigates compliance with these requirements if violations are alleged. Plans operating in states seeking to require enrollment of Medicaid beneficiaries in managed care were subject to specific federal rules governing such programs. While changes made by the Balanced Budget Act of 1997 now permit states to require enrollment in a managed care plan without obtaining prior federal approval, the new law also includes more extensive federal requirements for Medicaid managed-care plans.

HCFA also is responsible for issuing regulations applying the requirements of the Health Insurance Portability and Accountability Act of 1996 to "health insurance issuers." HMOs and PPOs are treated as issuers under HIPAA, except when they function as third-party administrators or perform other roles that do not involve the transfer of risk from a group plan to the HMO or PPO. HIPAA gives states the opportunity to enforce the new federal law for insured products and limits direct HHS involvement in this market to cases in which a state declines the opportunity to enforce the statute or fails substantially to enforce a particular HIPAA requirement.

The Department of Labor is the federal agency with primary responsibility for administering ERISA, including recent amendments made by HIPAA. DOL's principal regulatory role to date has been to assure that individuals who have employment-based health-care coverage are provided adequate notice of the terms and conditions of their coverage and that plan sponsors deliver promised benefits. To this end, ERISA imposes various documentation, reporting, and disclosure requirements and preempts state laws (other than state laws that regulate insurance) that "relate to" such plans.

Until the recent changes made by HIPAA, the ERISA statute did not generally regulate the content of these plans. Although ERISA does not directly regulate health insurance issuers, its requirements for employment-based plans frequently shape what plan sponsors expect from the health plans with which they contract.

The Office of Personnel Management administers the Federal Employees Health Benefits Program (FEHBP), which provides health benefits coverage to federal employees, retirees, and dependents and is the largest employer-sponsored health plan in the nation. Like Medicare, FEHBP sets threshold standards that plans must meet in order to participate in the program. The standards are intended to assure that plans have sufficient financial resources, experience, and network capacity to accommodate enrollment from FEHBP.

The Department of Defense administers the military health services system (MHSS), which provides medical care to active duty military personnel, their families, and retirees not yet eligible for Medicare. Although its budget is substantial, MHSS is not yet a major force in the regulation of HMOs and PPOs due to the structure of its managed-care contracting initiatives and the limited number of contractors involved in its programs.

State Regulation

Health plans often are regulated by more than one state agency—usually the department of insurance (which generally oversees the financial aspects of health plan operations) and the department of health (which generally regulates the health-care delivery system, including oversight on access and quality of care). Because states are also purchasers of health care for their own employees and through Medicaid programs, other state agencies also may be involved in setting standards for HMOs.

States are assisted in the task of regulating prepaid plans by the National Association of Insurance Commissioners, which drafted an HMO Model Act in 1972 and has updated it periodically. Building on the precedent set for other types of insurance, the model act requires prepaid plans to obtain a license in order to operate in a state, and it conditions issuance of the license on compliance with various requirements. In addition, the NAIC has developed numerous model acts and regulations that serve as the basis for state action in a significant number of areas, such as quality assurance, utilization review, and grievances and appeals. While the model acts encourage some general uniformity in the state regulation of HMOs, the details of licensure and other requirements frequently vary from state to state.

There is also an NAIC model act for preferred provider arrangements. Many states have opted to regulate PPOs through the insurance code or through stand-alone legislation that often addresses the activities performed by a PPO, such as utilization review.

Private Regulation

Independent accrediting organizations also set standards for HMOs and PPOs, and although these standards do not have the force and effect of law, they often play a significant role in shaping key aspects of plan design and operations. Increasing numbers of large employers and other purchasers are seeking external validation of the health plans with which they contract. Many state HMO laws explicitly recognize private accreditation; a few even require it. Recent changes in federal law have paved the way for Medicare to take into consideration private accreditation of quality assurance programs in determining whether comparable federal standards have been met.

Areas of Regulation

Health-plan regulators have addressed a number of aspects of plan operations, including quality assurance and utilization review, solvency, benefits, enrollment rules, enrollee information, access to care, provider contracting, premiums and rating practices, grievances and appeals, management and organizational structure, reporting and disclosure, and confidentiality. Since regulatory authority is dispersed among various agencies and organizations, health plans must often comply with multiple standards in each of these areas.

Quality Assurance and Utilization Review

Although it is difficult to draw a line between quality assurance activities and other aspects of HMO operations, this chapter includes four major topics under this rubric: provider credentialing, quality assurance programs, utilization review, and external review for quality of care.

Typically, plans must have quality assurance programs that reflect their activities in monitoring quality, assessing any quality problems, imposing corrective actions, and analyzing patterns of care. Also, plans frequently are required to involve physicians in establishing the program and reviewing the care process. In addition, plans may be required to have contracts with external organizations to review the quality of care.

Solvency

Solvency standards are intended to assure that health plans have sufficient resources to provide promised benefits. Although solvency standards differ from one regulatory program to another, most regulators require HMOs and PPOs to meet such standards and to update financial data periodically.

Benefits

Federal and state officials have adopted policies requiring health plans to provide specified benefits, either as a condition of receiving a contract under a federal or state health-care program, as a condition of state licensure, or to comply with a separate legal mandate. Some jurisdictions also have adopted policies that, while stopping short of an outright mandate, require health plans to comply with certain requirements if they offer a particular benefit.

Enrollment Rules

Regulators have established two types of rules regulating enrollment in health plans: those specifying a process (e.g., open enrollment) and those limiting the grounds on which plans may exclude an individual.

Enrollee Information

Virtually every entity that sets standards for health plans requires the plans to provide detailed information to enrollees and prospective enrollees about various aspects of health plan policies and operations. Increasingly, purchasers of health benefits are asking for comparative information.

Access to Care

Because many health plans provide benefits primarily through networks of providers, it has become increasingly common for regulators to set standards to measure the adequacy of these networks (i.e., to determine whether there are enough providers to furnish covered services to an enrolled population without undue delays). There also have been efforts to regulate other aspects of access, such as member choice of providers and direct access to providers.

Provider Contracting

HMO and PPO regulators generally have imposed three different kinds of requirements relating to health plan contracts with providers. Some have required HMOs to disclose to regulators the contents, or to report on certain aspects, of their provider contracts, often as a way of permitting regulators to monitor compliance. A second kind requires contracts to include (or to not include) certain substantive provisions. A third kind of regulation addresses the process that plans use to select the providers with which they contract.

Premiums and Rating Practices

Health plan premiums affect the costs incurred by purchasers, the pool of funds available for covered benefits, and the out-of-pocket costs of enrollees. Because of this, regulatory oversight of plan premiums is substantial.

Grievances and Appeals

Regulators generally require health plans to have internal grievance and appeals processes to resolve enrollee complaints against the organization. Typically, they also distinguish between the level of review that is provided for relatively minor complaints and for complaints about determinations that deny, reduce, or terminate benefits. Some plans, including Medicare and a few states plans, require independent external review of certain adverse plan determinations resulting in a denial of coverage or payment.

Management and Organizational Structure

Regulatory requirements regarding a health plan's management and organizational structure fall into three main categories. Some are intended to assure clear accountability for plan policies by easily identifiable individuals. Others are intended to assure the involvement of individuals with appropriate expertise and experience in specific decision-making areas (e.g., physician involvement in the development of practice guidelines). Still others are intended to exclude from HMO management individuals with a conflict of interest or with prior convictions for health care–related offenses.

Reporting and Disclosure

Health plans often must comply with extensive information reporting requirements—particularly in the areas of solvency and quality assurance—and provide reasonable access to actual plan records to permit verification of reported information. Sometimes this information is used to monitor continuing compliance with applicable standards; in other instances, it is used as the basis for consumer information.

Confidentiality

Health plans are required to comply with applicable state and federal laws intended to protect the confidentiality of information about the health status and treatment of identifiable individuals. Some also establish standards for assuring prompt access by patients to their own medical records and the accuracy of information contained in such records.

Other Areas

Health plans also must comply with federal, state, and local laws of general applicability. For example, health plans must be organized under state law, which usually means that they must apply for incorporation under the corporations law of a state and must meet whatever requirements that entails. Likewise, they must meet applicable state and local health and safety standards, zoning laws, and certificate of need requirements.

In addition, some states have established "claims" settlement laws governing the process and time frames by which insurers must process and pay claims. Finally, health plans must comply with civil rights or antidiscrimination laws, which affect all aspects of their operations, including hiring, contracting, and enrollment practices as well as product design.

Key Findings: The Impact of Four Managed-Care Legislative Proposals on Households, Employers, and Governments

A number of legislative proposals have been introduced at the state and federal levels that would affect the operation of health-care plans. The American Association of Health Plans commissioned Barents Group LLC to analyze four specific types of legislation affecting managed-care plans. For each type of provision, Barents estimated the effect on managed-care plan premiums and the effect of such premium increases on businesses, households, and governments. The Barents Group's findings are contained in its final report, entitled "Impacts of Four Legislative Provisions on Managed Care Consumers: 1999–2003."

Impact of Specific Provisions

The following four provisions were analyzed:

- increasing the exposure of health plans to malpractice liability;
- deeming utilization review to be part of the practice of medicine;
- prohibiting health plans from playing a role in making medical necessity determinations when making coverage decisions; and
- requiring plans to allow any willing provider into their network if the provider meets certain qualifications and is willing to abide by plan requirements.

The relative impact of each provision depends on a number of factors, including how the provision affects the ability of plans to efficiently manage utilization and to negotiate discounts from providers and also the level of additional direct costs health plans incur. For each provision, Barents estimated the provision's impact on managed-care plan costs (in percentages) by reviewing available literature and also working with an expert panel of actuaries, health plan legal counsel, and health plan medical directors to develop consensus judgments.[1] The panel members' expertise in the day-to-day operations and costs of managed-care plans provided additional perspectives in developing cost estimates. Using a variety of national and regional data sources, Barents developed models to estimate the financial impact of these cost increases, above current baseline projections, on households, businesses, and government.[2]

Impact of Provisions Affecting Liability of Health Plans

Barents estimates a premium increase of between 2.7 percent and 8.6 percent. With such premium increases, if employers absorb all of the cost increases, Barents projects a potential wage loss of between $475 and $1,512 per covered household from 1999 to 2003 as wages are reduced to offset higher premiums.

Alternatively, if managed-care cost increases are shared by employers and employees, these cost increases are projected to:

- increase total employment-based spending by between $38.7 billion and $123.1 billion for private firms, households, and state and federal governments from 1999 to 2003;
- increase costs by between $109 and $346 per covered household from 1999 to 2003;
- decrease employment by between 75,200 and 239,500 in 2003; and
- decrease the number of insured individuals by between 561,300 and 1.8 million in 1999.[3]

Impact of Provisions Defining Utilization Review as Practice of Medicine

Barents estimates a premium increase of between 2.2 percent and 6.9 percent. With such premium increases, if employers absorb all of the cost increases, Barents projects a potential wage loss of between $411 and $1,290 per covered household from 1999 to 2003 as wages are reduced to offset higher premiums.

Alternatively, if managed-care cost increases are shared by employers and employees, these cost increases are project to:

- increase total employment-based spending by between $33.5 billion and $104.9 billion for private firms, households, and state and federal governments from 1999 to 2003;
- increase costs by between $93 and $291 per covered household from 1999 to 2003;
- decrease employment by between 70,000 and 219,500 in 2003; and
- decrease the number of insured individuals by between 519,800 and 1.6 million in 1999.[4]

Impact of Provisions Related to Determining Medical Necessity for Purposes of Making Coverage Decisions

Barents estimates a premium increase of between 4.1 percent and 6.1 percent. With such premium increases, if employers absorb all of the cost increases, Barents projects a potential wage loss of between $749 and $1,124 per covered household from 1999 to 2003 as wages are reduced to offset higher premiums.

Alternatively, if managed-care cost increases are shared by employers and employees, these cost increases are projected to:

- increase total employment-based spending by between $62.9 billion and $94.5 billion for private firms, households, and state and federal governments from 1999 to 2003;
- increase costs by between $191 and $286 per covered household from 1999 to 2003;
- decrease employment by between 127,700 and 191,500 in 2003; and
- decrease the number of insured individuals by between 946,800 and 1.4 million in 1999.[5]

Impact of Provisions Related to Any Willing Provider

Barents estimates a premium increase of between 6.6 percent and 8.6 percent. With such premium increases, if employers absorb all of the cost increases, Barents projects a potential wage loss of between $1,213 and $1,579 per covered household from 1999 to 2003 as wages are reduced to offset higher premiums.

Alternatively, if managed-care cost increases are shared by employers and employees, these cost increases are projected to:

- increase total employment-based spending by between $101.8 billion and $132.8 billion for private firms, households, and state and federal governments from 1999 to 2003;

- increase costs by between $307 and $403 per covered household from 1999 to 2003;
- decrease employment by between 206,700 and 269,000 in 2003; and
- decrease the number of insured individuals by between 1.5 million and 2 million in 1999.[6]

Barents Group used a number of public and private data sources to analyze the impact of higher health-care costs for businesses, households, and governments. Estimates of total health insurance premiums, for example, were derived from recent Congressional Budget Office projections. Estimates on the number of individuals enrolled in various types of health plans were based on data filed with state regulators by health plans and surveys conducted by the National Research Corporation. Other data sources used in the analysis included the Current Population Survey (CPS), the Barents Business Model, and the Regional Economic Models Incorporated (REMI) model of national and state economies. Key assumptions, such as the extent to which employers lower wages as a result of higher employment costs, were developed using existing economic and health services research.

Barents Group LLC is a wholly owned subsidiary of KPMG Peat Marwick, one of the largest and most diversified professional services firms in the world. Barents Group is a leader in providing economic and financial advisory services to governments, philanthropic foundations, corporations, and associations. For its diversified client base, Barents' Health Economics Practice provides health services research, cost estimation, legislative analysis, strategic and operational assistance, and advisory services related to health sector reform.

NOTES

1. For modeling purposes only, cost increases were assumed to be limited to managed-care plans. To produce conservative estimates, indemnity plan costs were assumed not to be affected by the provisions themselves or by any "spillover" effect of increased managed-care plan costs.

2. The estimated impacts understate the effects of these provisions because managed-care plans' 1996 market share (about 70 percent of employer-sponsored health coverage) was used in this analysis. Market-share data from 1996 were used since sufficient detail was available to support state-level analysis. Because managed-care plans now account for about 85 percent of all employer-sponsored coverage and their market share is likely to continue growing, the use of 1996 market-share data produces conservative estimates of the effects of these legislative proposals.

3. The report contains a range estimate. At the high end of the range, 2.4 million individuals lose coverage.

4. The report contains a range estimate. At the high end of the range, 2.2 million individuals lose coverage.

5. The report contains a range estimate. At the high end of the range, 1.9 million individuals lose coverage.

6. The report contains a range estimate. At the high end of the range, 2.7 million individuals lose coverage.

PART 4

The Role of Regulation and Litigation

CHAPTER 12

The Role of State Insurance Regulators

Frances Wallace

States have been involved in regulating managed-care plans since their inception. Blue Cross Blue Shield Plans, which were arguably the first PPO plans, became subject to state insurance regulation soon after their creation. In the 1970s, as HMOs became more common, some states required them to be licensed as health facilities or agencies under statutes that also regulated them as insurance-risk-bearing entities. As health insurers began adding managed-care elements to their policies during the 1980s, states added requirements to their insurance laws to address this development. States have regulated insurance to protect their citizens from financial loss due to insurer insolvencies and from deceptive and unfair underwriting, marketing, and claims payment practices. They have also regulated to improve access to and affordability of health insurance coverage in the small employer and individual health insurance markets.

The federal government has also been involved with the health insurance marketplace. In 1973, Congress, through passage of the HMO Act, encouraged the development of HMOs by preempting state law restrictions on the corporate practice of medicine and prepaid group practices and by requiring certain employers to offer HMO coverage as part of their employee benefit plans. In 1974, with the passage of ERISA, Congress preempted all state laws that relate to employer-based health plans, except state laws that regulate the business of insurance, banking, or securities. Employers have responded to ERISA by self-funding their health plans to avoid state benefit and provider mandates, as well as state unfair claim practice and punitive damage statutes and state premium taxes. ERISA removed state authority to regulate the content of self-funded employer health plans, their financial solvency, or their contractual relationships with providers and did not replace it with federal laws regulating those same areas. The federal government has also used its role as a purchaser of health care for Medicare, Medicaid, and federal employees to indirectly regulate the behavior of insurers in the private health insurance market.

State insurance regulators recognize the increasing federal role in managed-care insurance regulation. Since the enactment of ERISA in 1974, states have been able to regulate health insurance mainly in the individual and small employer markets, which account for somewhere between 15 to 50 percent of private health-care coverage, depending upon the state.[1] States recognize that because of ERISA only the federal government can regulate the behavior of self-funded employers in the health-care marketplace. Although the federal role in managed-care regulation has increased, states can still play a role in the health-care marketplace, by concentrating their efforts in areas where they can have the most impact. These areas are likely to be those that focus on the regulation of the finances of managed-care plans, regulation of MCO processes and procedures, regulation of information, regulation of benefits, and regulation of risk relationships between MCOs and contracted providers.

States are likely to be less successful in legislating benefit and provider access mandates because of ERISA preemption. Because of federal preemption, state benefit and provider access mandates do not affect over half of the health insurance market. Additional state mandates will only encourage more employers to choose self-funding to avoid them. State benefit or provider access mandates may be more successful when limited to small employer and individual health insurance purchasers, since self-funding is not usually a viable option for most participants in these markets.

Areas of Regulation

In many states, insurance and health departments jointly regulate managed-care plans that are licensed as HMOs. Typically, insurance departments regulate HMO risk arrangements, financial reporting, pricing adequacy and equity, claims processing, and coverage documents and coverage determinations. Health departments oversee network adequacy, provider access and credentialing, and the assessment of quality assurance and improvement activities.[2] Usually state insurance departments have sole responsibility for regulating managed-care plans that are licensed as insurance companies or health-care service companies.

Regulation of Finances

Regulation of the solvency of insurance risk bearers is the one traditional state regulatory function that the federal government seems relatively likely to leave with the states. Concern in Congress about the adequacy of state financial regulation of insurance companies, including managed-care companies, has eased since state insurance departments have strengthened their solvency regulation through adoption of the accreditation program proposed by the National Association of Insurance Commissioners. From 1990 through 1998, forty-nine states have had their financial regulatory programs accredited by the NAIC.[3]

State regulators and state legislators are also developing new approaches to solvency regulation that can be applied to newly emerging categories of managed-care plans, for example, physician hospital organizations, provider service networks (PSNs), provider sponsored organizations, and integrated service delivery networks (ISDNs). Minnesota and Iowa have passed licensure laws that apply specifically to provider service organizations that bear insurance risk.[4] Ohio passed the Managed Care Uniform Licensure Act, which sets different levels of solvency regulation based upon how a managed-care entity functions in the marketplace.[5] The willingness of states to adopt solvency regulation that accomplishes the basic goal of protecting consumers without being unduly burdensome to new types of organizations should limit the push by the organizations for federal preemption.

One example of the federal-state balance in this area involves the implementation of the federal waivers of state licensure for Medicare + Choice Provider Sponsored Organizations required by the Balanced Budget Act of 1997. HCFA negotiated rules for federal PSO waivers with representatives of health care providers, health plans, and state regulators. The resulting rules set fairly high financial standards for federally waived PSOs, with the result that through the end of 1998 only three PSOs had applied for federal waivers of state managed-care licensure requirements.[6]

Regulation of Processes and Procedures

Insurance regulators have realized that most health benefit plans, regardless of the corporate form or licensing status of the risk bearer, incorporate some basic elements that are commonly considered managed care. Most insured health-care consumers are in plans that either require or encourage them to receive services from health-care facilities and providers that have contracts with the health plan. Most insured health-care consumers are also covered by plans that require some degree of prior authorization by the health plan for at least some high-cost medical services. When health plans require or encourage their enrollees to use providers that the health plan chooses for them, enrollees expect that someone is making sure that the health plan contracts with an adequate number of providers and monitors the quality of those providers. When health plans are able to deny delivery of or payment for services that an enrollee believes to be covered benefits, enrollees expect to have effective mechanisms for challenging those denials. Based on these expectations, insurance regulators, through the NAIC, have developed five model laws that address quality assessment and improvement as well as provider credentialing and standards of network adequacy; in addition, the models also propose a mechanism for providers to challenge adverse utilization review decisions and for enrollees to challenge adverse coverage or service delivery determinations. If states enact statutes based on these models, there would be a uniform approach to the regulation of certain basic managed-care elements that consumers tend to expect state insurance departments to handle. Although states could not apply the consumer protections in these models to most self-funded employer health plans, the enactment of these protections is not as likely as benefit mandates, for example, to be perceived by employers as a burden to be avoided and, therefore, is not likely to encourage more employers to self-fund health benefit plans.

Insurance regulators are typically the most concerned with processes and procedures that enable prospective purchasers and policyholders to challenge insurers when they refuse to issue or continue insurance and when they deny or limit insurance benefits. Even though state statutes allow policyholders to sue their insurers over claim denials, most states do not rely entirely on such private enforcement to protect their citizens from unfair insurance trade practices. Most states have unfair trade practice statutes that provide for administrative action by the insurance regulator in cases where insurers mislead policyholders about coverage or unfairly limit or deny claims. All state insurance regulators also have staff members who assist consumers in resolving complaints against insurers. Such consumer assistance serves an important public function to the extent that it helps to restore and preserve consumer trust in the insurance system. This is especially important as it applies to health insurance. Our system relies on private health insurance to provide access to health care for as many citizens as possible, principally through employer-sponsored health plans. Covered individuals need to be able to interact effectively with their health plans to get the benefits promised to them through their insurance contract. Since the interest of the employers who purchase the group health insurance contracts may sometimes run counter to the interests of their employees who actually use the benefits under those contracts, employers cannot necessarily be relied upon to advocate for their employees when the group insurer denies benefits.

With the advent of managed care, health insurers have more incentive to deny a claim before a service is delivered than they did when they were only writing unmanaged traditional indemnity policies. Under unmanaged indemnity policies, an insured would file a claim with an insurer after a service had been delivered, and any dispute about the cost of that service and the medical necessity for it was between the health-care provider and the insurer. Managed-care policies require preauthorization of many services: whether a service is a covered benefit is decided before the service is rendered. Denials of claims become denials of care. In such a situation, it is imperative that a managed-care plan enrollee be able to challenge a decision to deny care in a much more efficient manner than is afforded through the civil courts or even through administrative proceedings within state agencies. Consequently, most state managed-care statutes require plans to have an internal grievance procedure for handling such complaints in a relatively timely manner. If the enrollee is dissatisfied with the result of the internal process, he or she can appeal to a state agency.

As more citizens have experienced managed care, states have been motivated to expand and strengthen enrollee appeal rights against all types of health plans that have managed-care elements. Many states have passed laws that require all types of health insurers to provide enrollees with an expedited appeal in cases of life-threatening denials of care. Texas passed a law establishing a system for independent review of adverse benefit determinations by managed-care plans, but the United States Court of Appeals for the Fifth Circuit held that state-law requirements for external review were preempted by ERISA.[7] A petition for certiorari has been filed. If the Fifth Circuit opinion is upheld by the United States Supreme Court, it will significantly curtail state efforts in this area.

Regulation of Information

Regulation that addresses the information asymmetries between suppliers and consumers of all types of insurance, including health insurance, has long been an accepted role for state insurance regulators. Such regulation is consonant with the current emphasis on allowing the competitive market to determine the distribution and price of health insurance and regulating only to correct market imperfections. A common set of reporting requirements and publicly available health plan–level data is essential to a quality-based, competitive health-care market and can probably best be established by the government at the state and national level.

State insurance regulators already require detailed financial reporting from insurers in a format that is standardized across states, and they make this information available to the public. This helps purchasers make informed decisions about the financial strength of various insurers. State insurance laws also often require insurers and their agents to disclose certain types of information to potential purchasers and to current policyholders so that they can make better informed decisions when purchasing and using insurance coverage. Under managed care, information about the credentials of providers associated with particular health plans, and the medical outcomes that those plans achieve, becomes of much greater importance to consumers, since, unlike traditional health insurance, they have less choice in where they can seek medical care. As states have legislated financial reporting and information disclosure requirements for managed-care plans, they have often placed the responsibility for the administration of these laws with state insurance departments.

Information about the quality of service delivered by insurers has traditionally been available from state insurance departments only in the form of information about the number of complaints or market conduct administrative actions against insurers in given markets. Consumers need to know more than this to judge the quality of a managed-care plan. As a result, state insurance and managed-care regulators are beginning to provide more information in the form of health plan report cards that show standardized information about the types of care and the qualifications of providers so that consumers can compare health plans on the basis of quality as well as of price and solvency.

The biggest challenge in administering such requirements is to assure that the information is available to purchasers in a form that will actually encourage them to use it. This is especially true of information about the quality of managed-care plans. HEDIS is a set of quality of care measurements originally developed by private employers and later adopted by government payers such as Medicaid. HEDIS measures are widely available, yet recent studies have found that only about 6 percent of employers use HEDIS data to help them select managed-care plans and only 1 percent of employers make HEDIS data available to their employees.[8]

Regulation of Benefits

State insurance laws often require insurers to receive insurance department approval of their policies before they can market them to the public. State regulators review the policies not only to be sure that they contain any legislatively mandated coverages but also to determine that the policies clearly state what they do and do not cover, so that a potential purchaser can know with reasonable certainty what benefits the insurance will deliver when needed.

Mandated benefit laws result from the efforts of insurance purchasers and providers of services covered by insurance to get state legislatures to enact laws that require insurance policies to cover certain goods or services that they need or provide. This has been especially true of traditional health insurance and has carried over into managed-care policies. Because of ERISA preemption, state insurance benefit mandates only affect the underwritten customers of managed-care plans, usually just individuals and employers that are too small to self-insure, about one-third of the private market for health insurance. Only the federal government can mandate benefits for self-funded employer health plans. It has recently begun to do so, beginning with a mandate to cover hospital stays of at least forty-eight hours for new mothers.

As the federal government becomes more concerned with the content of health benefit plans offered through employers, they may want to structure laws in this area to take advantage of traditional state insurance department expertise in the content of insurance policies. The Medigap Improvements Act of 1990 and the Health Insurance Portability and Accountability Act of 1996 provide models of how federal-state cooperation might work. The Medigap Act requires private insurers to comply either with state laws that meet federal standards or with federal regulations where states fail to enact acceptable laws with regard to the content and marketing of Medigap insurance policies.[9] HIPAA requires health insurers and self-funded employer health plans to comply either with state laws that limit the application of preexisting condition exclusions in ways that meet federal standards or with HIPAA's "fallback" provisions.

Regulation of Provider–Health Plan Relationships

As managed care has become the dominant form of health insurance, health-care providers have lost the broad access to insured patients that they enjoyed when most people had traditional indemnity insurance. Consequently, providers have urged state legislatures to enact any willing provider laws. These laws require health insurers that condition the delivery of benefits upon the use of a particular panel of providers to accept into those panels any provider who is willing to accept the insurer's contracted level of reimbursement. Where states have enacted such laws, they have frequently been preempted by ERISA.

States have less of a problem with ERISA preemption when they regulate the content of the contracts between health insurers and health-care providers with regard to solvency and policyholder protection. State managed-care laws often empower insurance departments to regulate the payment and risk arrangements between managed-care plans and their contracted providers as a way to ensure health plan solvency. They also permit states to require policyholder protections in participating provider contracts, such as to hold harmless provisions and prohibitions against gag clauses. Such traditional insurance regulatory functions are more likely to survive ERISA preemption challenges.

Conclusion

It seems clear that whatever form managed-care regulation takes in the years to come, it will have both state and federal government components. Experience with the Medigap Act and HIPAA has demonstrated that states can work cooperatively with the federal government to enact and administer laws that accomplish national objectives, while still allowing states the flexibility to experiment and respond to local circumstances. Administratively, it makes sense to use both state and federal resources, as insurance regulation becomes ever more federalized. States insurance and health departments have regulatory expertise in areas of managed care that are different from the traditional competencies of federal departments, such as the Department of Health and Human Services and the U.S. Department of Labor. By combining this expertise and learning to work together rather than in duplication, regulation of the health-care marketplace can be improved and strengthened.

NOTES

1. *Databook on Employee Benefit Plans,* 5th ed. Washington, D.C. (Employee Benefit Research Institute, 1997), 35–52.

2. "The Regulation of Health Plans," American Association of Health Plans, Feb. 3, 1998, p. 11.

3. John K. Iglehart, "State Regulation of Managed Care: NAIC President Josephine Musser," *Health Affairs* 16 (1997): 38.

4. Allison Overby and Mark Hall, "Insurance Regulation of Providers that Bear Risk," *American Journal of Law and Medicine* 22 (1996): 361–410.

5. Ohio Department of Insurance Policy Statement on the Managed Care Uniform Licensure Act (S.B. 67) and the Regulation of Risk-Bearing Entities, p. 1.

6. 42 CFR 422.350–422.384, as listed in the Federal Register, June 26, 1998, 63 (123):35098–99 at http://www.hcfa.gov/medicare/mtcreg3.pdf.

7. *Corporate Health Insurance, Inc. v. Texas Department of Insurance,* 220 F. 3d 641 (5th Cir. 2000), petition for certiorari filed (2001).

8. "Employers, Employees Don't Use Plan Data," *Modern Healthcare* 40, September 21, 1998.

9. Margaret G. Farrell, "ERISA Preemption and Regulation of Managed Health Care: The Case for Managed Federalism," *American Journal of Law and Medicine* 23 (1997): 287–88.

CHAPTER 13

The Role of Private Litigation in Monitoring Managed Care

Peter D. Jacobson

During the past decade, health-care delivery has been evolving away from a system in which individual physicians provide care for individual patients toward a system characterized by large patient populations within integrated delivery systems. Perhaps the most dominant social force behind this transformation has been the need to contain the rising cost of delivering health-care services.

The success of these recent changes, especially the cost-containment initiatives introduced by managed-care organizations, depends largely on whether the cost-containment efforts and other managed-care innovations can lower health-care costs without reducing quality of care. Yet, the ability to sustain and expand those innovations also depends on how courts decide litigation challenging these innovations. If courts consistently rule in favor of individual patients' service delivery needs, it may be difficult to sustain cost-control mechanisms. But if courts consistently rule in favor of cost containment, individuals will have little recourse when medical care is denied. Judicial decisions will also influence the expansion of the new organizational forms and physician autonomy.

In responding to the litigation, judges face a threshold question of what role courts should play in monitoring the managed-care environment relative to legislatures. Courts face the tension of applying common law liability principles to new situations (perhaps by depicting public policy considerations) or deferring to elected representatives to set public policy. In the new health-care environment, courts will be asked to distinguish the economic aspects of managed care that order relationships among health plans, physicians, and patients from the incentives that contribute to below-standard care. The former are more traditionally legislative prerogatives while the latter are traditionally within the judicial purview. The evolution of both common law and constitutional law is replete with examples of this tension, with courts expanding liability principles in some instances (such as imposing strict liability for mass-produced goods) and deferring to the legislatures in others (such as with physician-assisted suicide).

This chapter provides an initial assessment of how the courts have ruled in private litigation affecting managed-care cost-containment initiatives.[1] By cost-containment initiatives, I mean that set of managed-care practices designed to reduce the costs of health care, such as prospective utilization management, capitated funding arrangements, limitations on choice of providers, and other incentives (e.g., bonuses and withholds) that encourage providers to limit medical treatment. The chapter addresses the role of private litigation in monitoring health plans' quality of care and in setting the liability context in holding plans accountable for their cost-containment initiatives. It will also assess the type of litigation that has emerged to date, how the courts have ruled, and what factors courts have considered in rendering judgments in managed-care cases. The presentation is organized around five interrelated questions:

- What are the emerging trends in managed-care liability?
- How are courts deciding challenges to cost-containment initiatives?
- Do courts understand the underlying changes in health-care delivery?
- Are courts deferring to the market, or is health care treated differently than other commodities?
- Are courts deferring to the legislatures to set public policy in managed care?

Taken together, the answers to these questions will enable stakeholders and policymakers to understand the courts' receptivity to changing circumstances and the flexibility with which MCOs will be allowed to operate. The analysis will provide an initial look at the development of legal doctrine in managed care, what policies legislators and regulators should consider in response, and how health-care delivery, especially physician autonomy, might be influenced by the emerging trends.

Private Litigation

The involvement of the courts in monitoring health care is not new. For many years, courts have been actively involved in monitoring quality of care through medical liability determinations by establishing the applicable standard of care (Jacobson 1989) and in interpreting the range of benefits to be provided through contractual determinations of what constitutes medical necessity (Hall and Anderson 1992; Eddy 1996). Courts have also been called upon to interpret the vast array of state and federal legislation regulating health-care delivery. What is new in the managed-care environment are the types of issues likely to emerge, particularly the conflict between population-based cost containment and access for individual subscribers, the multiplicity of actors in a given case, and the evolving nature of the organizational structures.

Both public law, defined as "That portion of the law that defines rights and duties with either the operation of government, or the relationships between government and individuals,"[2] and private law, usually thought of as litigation between private parties over contracts and torts (which are civil wrongs, such as negligence), will help shape the legal environment in which MCOs operate, though the distinction between the two is often blurred. For instance, while most of the cost-containment initiatives will be challenged and adjudicated as private law issues, public law involving Medicare and Medicaid will be important, as those programs shift their beneficiary coverage into MCOs. Private law will play a dominant role in shaping the liability environment (unless altered by state legislatures) that will help order private relationships among physicians, patients, and health-care plans.

Although some commentators have argued that the courts should make radical alterations in medical liability doctrine (Morreim 1989; Havighurst 1995; Abraham and Weiler 1994),[3] common law liability doctrine has traditionally emerged incrementally to adapt to changing circumstances (Hall 1989). This incremental approach to developing legal doctrine in a new industry (such as during the emergence of railroads in the nineteenth century) has the advantage of permitting the courts to maintain a dialogue with other courts and stakeholders and to adjust to changing circumstances, but it has the disadvantage of the lack of predictability. Even more troublesome is that the underlying changes in health-care delivery are occurring much more rapidly than the courts can respond.

Functions of Litigation

Traditionally, private civil litigation serves three basic purposes: compensation, deterrence, and accountability. At issue are the expected outcomes of private litigation: damages, internal policy changes by MCOs, or state or federal governmental changes in public policy. From a policy perspective, the ability of private litigation to achieve broad policy changes may be limited (Rosenberg 1991).

The most obvious function of the tort system is to compensate an injured victim for harm suffered as a result of the defendant's wrongdoing. Compensation includes economic damages (actual medical expenses, for instance) but can also include noneconomic damages for pain and suffering. This may be thought of as the law's corrective function and is determined through liability standards, as discussed later.

The second function of the tort system is to deter future wrongdoing. In medical liability litigation, deterrence would include attempts to diminish the likelihood of future deviations from the standard of care.

A closely related function is accountability. By establishing rules to assess liability, the tort system provides a mechanism for society to hold wrongdoers accountable for their actions. The accountability function will be especially important as the courts begin to assess the consequences and available remedies for aggressive cost-containment initiatives.

Establishing Medical Liability

To establish medical liability, an injured patient must show that the physician failed to exercise the appropriate standard of care owed to that patient. The patient must also prove that the failure to maintain the standard of care caused the injury and that damages were incurred. In medical liability cases, the medical profession sets its own standard of care based on what is customary and usual practice, as established through physician testimony and medical treatises. Courts are reluctant to substitute their judgment for that of the medical profession, even when a new, safer technology is being considered (Jacobson and Rosenquist 1988; Jacobson 1989).

Each physician must exercise the degree of skill ordinarily practiced, under similar circumstances, by members of the profession. Physicians with special knowledge, such as cardiologists, will be held to customary practices among those of similar skill and training. If, however, there is more than one recognized course of treatment, most courts allow some flexibility in what is regarded as customary treatment, known as the respectable minority rule.

Health care institutions, including MCOs, may also be held liable for the negligence of their employees, either under a theory of direct liability or under agency principles (vicarious liability). As a general rule, health-care institutions may be held liable for the failure to (1) maintain safe and adequate facilities, (2) select and retain competent physicians, (3) oversee all patient care within the institution, and (4) ensure quality care (*McClellan v. HMO of Pennsylvania*, 604 A.2d 1053 (Pa.Super. 1992)).

ERISA Preemption

At the outset, it is necessary to consider the dominant role played by ERISA in shaping the current managed-care litigation context. According to recent Department of Labor estimates, ERISA applies to approximately 125 million Americans covered by employer-sponsored health plans.[4] ERISA plans include those that are self-funded by the employer and those where the employer purchases health-care coverage from a third-party insurer. At the risk of oversimplifying a very complex statute, the ability of ERISA-covered managed-care subscribers to sue an MCO depends primarily on how courts interpret ERISA's preemption provision. In this context, preemption means that state laws (including legislation and court decisions) purporting to regulate health plans may not be enforced in any court. Because ERISA permits recovery only for the amount of a claimed benefit, the practical consequence of successfully invoking ERISA preemption is to insulate MCOs from exposure to monetary damages. (Those not covered by ERISA have no similar litigation constraints.)

ERISA preempts all state laws (including state common law) that "relate to" an employee benefit plan (EBP). Broadly speaking, any law or legal action that requires the plan administrator to interpret the plan's benefits triggers preemption. For example, if a court rules that the MCO action being challenged relates to a benefits determination, such as the denial of additional hospital coverage, state litigation will be preempted because that action would require an interpretation of the plan's benefits.

Until recently, courts have interpreted the phrase "relates to" very broadly, preempting most challenges to health plan innovations and medical decisions. For instance, courts have consistently held that challenges to delayed or denied care relate to an EBP and are preempted.[5] But recent cases have established the principle that challenges to the technical quality of care (i.e., liability claims for substandard clinical care) do not involve the administration of plan benefits and will not be preempted, allowing state courts to resolve the liability allegations.[6] Challenges to the quantity of care (involving plan benefit decisions) will still be preempted, hence protecting cost-containment practices. In practice, the quantity-quality distinction is difficult to maintain, as many clinical decisions involve both aspects. For instance, discharging a patient two days early may represent a clinical decision or it may be based on a benefits determination.

The broader the scope of ERISA preemption, the greater the leeway for MCOs to implement cost-containment initiatives. Challenges to delayed or denied care resulting from cost-containment initiatives will usually involve an interpretation of plan benefit decisions and are therefore vulnerable to ERISA preemption. Thus, the first hurdle in challenging managed-care cost-containment programs is whether courts will preempt the litigation altogether.

Liability Trends

To date, there have been relatively few decisions interpreting the extent of MCO medical liability. There are two primary reasons for this. First, the organizational changes toward managed care are relatively new. The full scope of cost-containment initiatives may not yet have been implemented, cases may be slowly emerging through the court system,[7] or disputes may have been decided through arbitration. Second, MCOs serving self-insured firms have relied on ERISA to preempt medical liability claims in state courts. Depending on whether the courts continue to narrow ERISA preemption, more liability claims may begin to be heard in state courts.

Despite variation in the state cases decided to date, the trend appears to be that courts are applying traditional liability doctrine to the new organizational forms, including HMOs, IPAs, and PPOs (Furrow 1997). For staff or group model HMOs, the law had already developed holding them liable for torts (civil wrongs) committed by their employees. The primary issue is whether courts will apply indirect liability doctrine (i.e., vicarious liability and agency principles) to the other MCO organizational forms for malpractice committed by an independent physician.

In determining vicarious liability, the courts look to the MCO's control over the physician or how the plan markets its physicians. The greater the indicia of control and the more the plan markets the quality of its physician panel, the greater the likelihood that the MCO will be held vicariously liable. In the leading case of *Boyd v. Albert Einstein Medical Center* (547 A.2d 1229 (Pa. Super. 1988)), for example, the court held that an HMO could be found liable for an individual physician's medical malpractice because the patient reasonably believed that the HMO controlled the physician. The court rejected the plan's argument that it was not liable because the physician was an independent contractor, holding that the physician could still be the plan's agent with respect to the patient. A key element is whether the MCO has sufficient control, such as through utilization management arrangements, to override a physician's clinical decision (Furrow 1997).[8]

Cost-Containment Initiatives

As noted already, courts are likely to exert a significant influence over the ability of MCOs to sustain and expand cost-containment initiatives. Several previous commentators have argued that the courts would most likely frustrate managed-care cost-containment initiatives. For example, Hall (1988) assessed similar initiatives adopted by hospitals (largely in a fee-for-service context) in the 1980s and the courts' responses to prior authorization, physician payment incentives, and physician selection, concluding that cost-containment innovations would not survive judicial scrutiny. Similarly, Anderson (1992) argued that courts have expanded their influence over health policy by, for example, overturning insurers' coverage decisions and favoring hospitals, as opposed to states, in Medicaid rate-setting cases under the Boren Amendment. Other commentators have also argued that courts have tended to side with individual patients against insurers in deciding whether expensive technologies are covered benefits (Ferguson, Dubinski, and Kirsch 1993).

In contrast, this chapter takes the position that to date there is no evidence that courts have systematically impeded cost-containment innovations. While it may be that many of the most challenging cost-containment innovations have yet to be litigated, there is evidence that courts are willing to uphold cost-containment initiatives.

Utilization Management

MCOs rely heavily on utilization management (UM) techniques to reduce costs. Courts have struggled with two interrelated aspects of utilization review: first, how to determine the locus of responsibility for inappropriate care; and second (discussed in a subsequent section), how to characterize utilization management under ERISA, as an insurance (benefits) determination or as a medical decision.

Despite uncertainty in how to characterize UM, courts have generally not impeded its use for containing costs, especially under ERISA. No court has ruled that UM programs violate public policy, and at least one court, *Varol v. Blue Cross & Blue Shield, Inc.* (708 F.Supp. 826 (E.D.Mich. 1989)), explicitly upheld a preauthorization arrangement. The fundamental issue is what happens when a UM firm or internal UM decision overrules the treating physician's clinical recommendation. Which entity should be held liable for any adverse consequences: the UM firm, the MCO, the treating physician, or a combination of these actors? In *Wilson v. Blue Cross of Southern California* (271 Cal.Rptr. 876 (Cal.Ct.App. 1990)), the California Supreme Court ruled that the UM firm should not be exempt from the consequences of its decisions and could be held liable if its decision was a substantial factor in causing a patient's injury. Previous California Supreme Court cases, however, had upheld the concept of retrospective review and coverage determinations.[9] Other courts have denied summary judgment to defendants, ruling that it would be a question of fact for the jury to determine whether UM decisions contributed to the adverse outcome.[10] The Wyoming Supreme Court recently extended this reasoning in permitting litigation against the UM firm to proceed, holding that the UM process involves medical decisions (*Long v. Great West Life & Annuity Insurance Company* (1998 Wyo. LEXIS 62)). Taken together, the reported non-ERISA UM cases establish no clear doctrine in allocating liability and demonstrate that the courts are uncertain in how to think about UM decisions.

It is likely that most of the future litigation involving UM will take place in the context of ERISA. The initial inquiry will be whether UM "relates to" the benefits plan or constitutes a medical determination. If the former is true, ERISA will preempt state liability challenges to adverse outcomes from the UM process. So far, federal courts have uniformly held that UM decisions relate to benefits plans and are preempted. For example, in *Jass v. Prudential Health Care Plan* (88 F.3d 1482 (7th Cir. 1996)), the court supported the prevailing view that a utilization review dispute was preempted by ERISA because it was a dispute over medical benefits, not medical care.[11]

Challenges to Capitation Arrangements

An issue that goes to the heart of managed-care cost-containment initiatives is whether a managed-care subscriber can sue his or her physician or health plan for negligence based on financially motivated clinical decisions. The theory used to challenge financial incentives is breach of fiduciary duty. At this point, no cases have actually determined liability based on financially motivated clinical decisions, and several cases have specifically rejected such challenges (see, e.g., *McClellan v. HMO of Pa.,* 604 A.2d 1053, 1056, footnote 6 (Pa. Super. 1992)).[12] Nevertheless, this area remains somewhat unsettled in view of two recent decisions and may be characterized as "watchful waiting"[13] while courts assess ongoing developments, such as health-care outcomes, based on financial incentives.

In *Paul v. Humana Medical Plan* (1996 WL 525518 (Fla.App. 4 Dist., 1996)), a Florida appellate court ruled that the plaintiff could sue a physician for negligence on the theory that financial considerations motivated the physician to deny referral to a specialist and to discharge the plaintiff prematurely from the hospital. And in *Pappas v. Asbel* (724 A.2d 889 (Pa. 1998), vacated and remanded for reconsideration in light of *Pegram v. Herdrich,* 120 S. Ct. 2686 (2000)), the court ruled that an HMO could be sued for negligence based on treatment delays allegedly caused by the HMO's cost-containment program. The court held that the alleged treatment delays do not relate to an ERISA benefits plan administration and are therefore not preempted. Liability has not been determined in either case—courts have simply allowed the cases to proceed to trial. But if these decisions are upheld and lead to jury awards, there will be a sustained attack on the foundation of financial incentives in other jurisdictions.[14]

Perhaps more important, in *Herdrich v. Pegram* (154 F.3d 362 (7th Cir. 1998), the court held that a patient could sue for breach of ERISA's fiduciary duty based on an allegation that the physician's economic incentives led to delayed care that resulted in an adverse outcome.* Although the *Herdrich* court specifically noted that the existence of economic incentives would not automatically be tantamount to a breach of fiduciary duty, this case is a potentially significant extension of the rationale advanced in other cases. If other courts follow and rule that the existence of economic incentives may constitute a breach of fiduciary duty challenge under ERISA, these incentives will be increasingly vulnerable to legal challenge (see, e.g., Morreim 1998).

Disclosure of Financial Incentives

A closely related cost-containment issue that has recently received considerable

---

*Editors' note: This case was reversed by the United States Supreme Court. Pegram v. Herdrich, 120 S. Ct. 2143 (2000). See chapter 3, note 10.

public attention is whether MCOs and physicians must disclose their financial incentives to patients. MCOs have argued vigorously that these economic incentives do not interfere with the exercise of their physicians' clinical judgment and should not be disclosed to patients. In two recent cases, courts have rejected this reasoning, allowing plan subscribers to sue for nondisclosure of economic incentives as a violation of ERISA's fiduciary duties (*Drolet v. Healthsource, Inc.,* No. CV-96-166-B (D.N.H. 1997); *Shea v. Esensten,* 107 F.3d 625 (8th Cir. 1997)). In *Shea,* the court held that the HMO's financial incentives, including incentives discouraging treatment referrals, were material facts that must be disclosed as part of ERISA's fiduciary duties.

Even if courts require the disclosure of economic incentives, this does not mean that courts are impeding cost-containment initiatives. It would only mean that those initiatives must be clearly communicated to patients, not that the incentives must be discontinued. Neither the *Drolet* nor the *Shea* court challenged the public policy legitimacy of the incentives themselves.[15] And in *Weiss v. Cigna Health Care, Inc.* (No. 96 Civ. 1107 (SHS), S.D.N.Y., July 23, 1997),[16] the court explicitly declined to follow the *Shea* and *Drolet* cases, holding that the claim "is tantamount to a claim that risk-sharing arrangements in managed care are inherently illegal, a position that is refuted by federal and New York law."

Physicians' Antitrust Challenges to Cost-Containment Programs

In the new health-care order, physicians have attempted to use antitrust doctrine through private litigation to block cost-containment initiatives, and competing organizations have attempted to use antitrust doctrine to force competitors to open their physician panels to competition. Neither effort has generated much support in the courts, as illustrated by two specific cases.

In *Ambroze v. Aetna Health Plans of New York, Inc.* (1996 WL 282069 (S.D.N.Y.), revised on other grounds, 107 F.3d 2 (2d Cir. 1997)), anesthesiologists brought a restraint of trade action under Section 1 of the Sherman Act, challenging the defendant's exclusive contracting arrangement with another physicians' group. After determining that a valid antitrust violation had not been alleged, the court attacked the heart of the plaintiffs' case. While not critical to the court's decision,[17] the court said "it is worth repeating the fact that the plaintiffs' principal target here . . . is the very concept of managed care. . . . The fact that HMOs have their critics . . . does not obligate the courts to create . . . a novel application of the antitrust laws. . . . [J]udicial restraint in this highly charged area of law and policy is the best recourse." On remand from the circuit court, in the now-titled case of *Finkelstein v. Aetna Health Plans of New York* (No. 95-CIV-6631 (DLC) (S.D.N.Y., July 1997)), the district court dismissed the plaintiffs' group boycott allegation, holding that Aetna could contract to purchase services from physicians at terms deemed mutually acceptable without incurring antitrust liability.

In *Blue Cross & Blue Shield of Wisconsin v. Marshfield* (65 F.3d 1406 (7th Cir. 1994)), the court considered the question of whether an HMO could use the antitrust laws to compel a competing organization (a physician-owned multispecialty clinic) to open its physician panel to competitors. The plaintiff argued that it could not compete for physicians' services in the area because the defendant controlled the physician market through exclusive contracting arrangements. Without access to the defendant's physician panel, the plaintiff could not contract with sufficient numbers of high-quality physicians to compete. The court held that the defendant's reputation for high-quality care allowed it to assure exclusivity, not any monopoly power. As such, the court refused to invoke antitrust principles to overturn exclusive relationships determined by market forces.

Understanding Changes in Health-Care Delivery

Not surprising, courts vary widely in their understanding of the underlying changes in health-care delivery. In areas such as antitrust, where judges can largely rely on traditional legal doctrine, courts have done fairly well. In other areas, such as utilization management, where they are dealing with an entirely new set of issues, the results have been mixed. One reason for this distinction is that in antitrust cases the courts have focused on operational details, such as the efficiencies of a given transaction, that can be applied to established legal principles. In other areas, especially in ERISA and utilization management cases, courts have focused on the form of the transaction instead of viewing functional or operational relationships, hence ignoring the nuances of a changing health-care environment.

There is, however, a learning curve at work. Some recent cases have rejected the MCOs' arguments for strictly separating clinical and financial functions, ruling instead that MCOs in fact make medical decisions.[18] The shifting understanding of how MCOs function may lead to closer judicial scrutiny of the MCOs' role in clinical decision making and hence greater difficulty in avoiding liability.

Facilitating Market-Based Arrangements

Several commentators have noted that antitrust doctrine has been an important contributor to the expansion of managed care (see, e.g., Havighurst 1995; Greaney 1994; Blumstein 1994).[19] By ruling that health care is not immune to antitrust considerations, starting with *Arizona v. Maricopa County Medical Society* (457 U.S. 332 (1982)), the courts opened the way to the new organizational arrangements. In general, courts have applied traditional antitrust principles to health-care markets (Greaney 1997), helping to stimulate the movement toward more efficient organizational forms. Recent merger decisions, along with the federal antitrust guidelines,[20] for instance, have focused on systems integration and economic efficiencies to determine whether an activity violates the antitrust laws.

A dramatic increase in the number of hospital mergers has been one of the characteristics of the new health-care order. As hospital bed occupancy has declined and as pressure from MCOs to reduce costs has intensified, hospitals have decided to merge to be in a better position to negotiate arrangements with MCOs. For the most part, the courts have been reluctant to interfere with this process. In several high-profile cases where the Department of Justice and the Federal Trade Commission have opposed mergers, courts have permitted them to proceed (*Federal Trade Commission v. Butterworth,* 946 F. Supp. 1285 (W.D.Mich. 1996); *United States v. Mercy Health Services,* 902 F. Supp. 968 (N.D.Iowa 1995)). While some of the specifics, such as permitting a seventy-three-mile primary care area in the *Mercy Health Services* case, have been controversial, courts have generally demonstrated that they understand the underlying market changes and have adapted traditional antitrust doctrine to those changes (Greaney 1997).

An important issue confronted by antitrust cases is how to characterize MCOs for purposes of defining the relevant product markets to analyze competition. Two recent cases have ruled that MCOs (either HMOs or IPAs) do not constitute a separate health-care market for antitrust analysis (*Blue Cross & Blue Shield of Wisconsin v. Marshfield,* 65 F.3d 1406 (7th Cir. 1994); *U.S. Healthcare, Inc. v. Healthsource, Inc.,* 986 F.2d 589 (1st Cir. 1993)), in part because physicians have other market alternatives for selling their services to insurers and MCOs. These cases indicate that courts are not protecting MCOs from competitive forces in the health-care market.

The Implications of New Organizational Forms and Arrangements

Courts have been less successful in understanding the implications of new organizational forms, particularly those such as IPAs and UM firms, which have mixed functions. In these cases, courts have more often viewed MCOs as mere financers of health care rather than understanding the MCOs' mixed functions as both insurer and provider. As a result, MCOs have been able to distance themselves somewhat from the full consequences of their actions as providers.

A particularly egregious example of the courts' failure to comprehend and respond to the changes in traditional organizational functions is the case of *McClellan v. HMO of Pennsylvania* (686 A.2d 801 (Pa. 1996)). The issue in this case was whether an IPA fell within the statutory definition of a health-care provider for purposes of a motion to compel the disclosure of certain documents. On a 3-to-3 tie vote, with one judge abstaining, the lower court's decision that an IPA did not meet the statutory definition of a health-care provider was upheld.

The judges voting for affirmance stated that "an IPA model is neither a direct health care practitioner, nor the administrator of a health care facility." In essence, these judges viewed the IPA strictly in relation to the older forms of health-care delivery, that "an IPA cannot be regarded as a health care provider because it cannot oversee patient care within its walls." In contrast, the three judges voting to characterize the IPA differently, and much more accurately, noted that the conclusion by the other judges

> ignores the reality of health care today. A corporation operating a health care facility . . . may not be in a place where it can oversee patient care "within its walls." More importantly, HMOs dictate the care provided in health care facilities. . . . Because HMOs manage patient care, they have the same duty as other health care facilities to select and retain competent physicians.

Utilization Management

As with new organizational forms, courts are struggling to characterize the combined functions of UM as a benefits determination and as a medical screen. In the ERISA context, as noted earlier, courts have generally defined UM narrowly as a benefits determination, even where medical care recommended by the treating physician is denied. For instance, in *Corcoran v. United Health Care, Inc.* (965 F.2d 1321 (5th Cir. 1992)), the court agreed with Corcoran that United's UM program involved clinical decisions and with United that part of its actions constituted a benefits determination. Concluding that United makes medical decisions in the context of determining benefits, the court preempted Corcoran's lawsuit under ERISA. The problem is that the court never explained what benefit was actually at issue, why United's action constituted a benefits determination, or why the aspect of the UM plan incident to a benefits decision should predominate over the clinical aspects.[21]

By characterizing the UM process as a benefits rather than clinical matter, the federal courts are providing wide latitude for health-care plans to control costs, at the possible expense of both individual access to health-care services and the treating physician's clinical autonomy. The ERISA cases supporting this analysis fail to analyze the legal significance of the mixed form of clinical and cost-containment decisions made through the UM process (Rosenblatt, Law, and Rosenbaum 1997). In these cases, courts have exalted form over function, ignoring the reality that UM represents a treatment decision that is incidental to an administrative benefit determination (Jacobson and Pomfret 1998). Just as it is largely impossible to separate an MCO's financing functions from its health-care delivery functions, the mixed functions served by UM cannot easily be disaggregated into separable decision processes.

Deference to the Market

Except for end-of-life cases, there is a good bit of evidence that courts treat health care as they would any other industry. Whether this amounts to deference to emerging market principles in health-care delivery remains to be seen. At a minimum, it suggests that courts will not reflexively overturn market decisions. The clearest evidence for this is in courts' increasing deference to contractual arrangements, in physicians' litigation against MCOs, and in antitrust cases where courts are not protecting MCOs from competitive forces in the health-care market. Arguably, one reason why cost-containment initiatives have not been overturned is that courts are looking to contract law to determine the extent of the parties' obligations and responsibilities. One area where the evidence of the shift to contract law is less clear is with decisions contesting benefits denials, particularly in life-threatening cases and in ERISA cases alleging a breach of fiduciary duties.

Deference to the Contract

For many years, some commentators, most prominently Professor Clark Havighurst, have been arguing that health-care delivery should be guided by market principles as determined through contractual arrangements (see, e.g., Havighurst 1995; Blumstein 1994; Morreim 1995; Hall 1997). In the most extreme form, contracts would be used to set all the parameters of the health-care relationship, including benefits determinations and liability standards. Most commentators adopt a less extreme contractual regime, where contracts would not establish all the terms of the relationship but would certainly be relied upon far more than courts have done in the past.

Physician Selection/Deselection

One area where courts have given MCOs wide authority to operate is in staff privileges, an area now dominated by contractual interpretations. MCOs have argued that one important aspect of controlling health-care costs is in limiting the number of physicians who are eligible to participate in the plan and in applying economic criteria to staff selection and retention decisions. For the most part, courts have sanctioned the use of economic credentialing and the use of selective contracting. In *Maltz v. Aetna Health Plans of New York* (114 F.3d 9 (2d Cir. 1997)), for example, the court upheld the MCO's change in network physicians based solely on cost-containment reasons despite the disruption to long-term physician-patient relationships. In this instance, physician-patient autonomy yielded to cost-containment dictates. Antitrust challenges to exclusive contractual arrangements as a group boycott have also failed.

Some courts, particularly in California, New Hampshire, and Pennsylvania, have imposed fair process requirements, including a fair hearing, as a condition of deselection. In *Potvin v. Metropolitan Life Insurance Company* (63 Cal.Rptr. 202 (Cal.Ct.App. 2d Dist. 1997)),[22] a case challenging termination from a provider network absent due process, the court cited previous California cases with approval that private organizations that control important economic interests attain a "quasi-public significance." Stating that the health plans in this case were "tinged with public stature or purpose," the court held that a fair hearing must be provided prior to termination. These courts have not gone beyond procedural requirements, suggesting that deselection may proceed in these jurisdictions once the procedural requirements have been satisfied. Similar procedural requirements in peer review determinations have not impeded hospitals from terminating staff privileges (see, e.g., Blum 1996). Indeed, courts have not yet held that clauses permitting termination without cause violate public policy, although one court has remanded the case for trial on that issue (*Harper v. Healthsource, Inc.,* 674 A.2d 962 (N.H. 1996)), another court overturned an arbitration panel's decision because the panel was not fair and impartial (*Rudolph v. Pennsylvania Blue Shield,* 717 A.2d 508 (Pa. 1998)), and at least one state, New York, has done so legislatively.

Arbitration Clauses

Two recent California cases interpreting Kaiser Permanente's arbitration provisions demonstrate both the willingness of courts to uphold contractual arrangements and some of the limits to contracting that courts may be willing to entertain. In *Toledo v. Kaiser Permanente Medical Group* (1997 U.S. Dist. LEXIS 3941 (N.D.Cal., 1997)), the court upheld Kaiser's arbitration provision against a challenge claiming that Kaiser did not adequately inform the plaintiff of the provision. Relying on the plaintiff's signature just below what the court termed a "clear and conspicuous" arbitration clause, the court rejected the challenge.

In *Engalla v. The Permanente Medical Group, Inc.* (No. S048811 (Cal.

1997)), the California Supreme Court refused to rule that the arbitration clause violates public policy (as inherently one-sided, or unconscionable, agreements) but allowed the plaintiff to avoid arbitration in this case because Kaiser's manipulation of the process prevented the arbitration from taking place in a timely manner. This case suggests that courts will be reluctant to overturn contractual provisions but will closely scrutinize how they are implemented to avoid unfairness or overreaching by MCOs.

Limitations

MCO cost-containment programs could be vulnerable to liability when patients sue to compel contractual coverage of certain medical interventions, such as high-cost or experimental treatments. A typical case might involve denial of high-dose chemotherapy, with autologous bone marrow transplant viewed as experimental. In a recent study, Hall et al. (1996)[23] found that treatment was ordered in 57 percent of the coverage cases reviewed. However, the sample included few managed care cases, and the authors found that treatment was ordered at a significantly lower rate in cases brought under ERISA. In addition, Morreim (1997, p. 46, n. 148) notes that courts in more recent non-ERISA cases have been less likely to rule in favor of patients, deferring instead to contractual arrangements limiting coverage. Nothing in more recent ERISA cases suggests that MCOs will be compelled to provide similar benefits. Thus, challenges to MCOs' coverage decisions are likely to be preempted by ERISA, though patients not covered by ERISA may have a better chance to compel treatment, depending on how the plan's contract is written.

The Courts and Public Policy

The cases decided so far suggest that courts will not systematically impede the implementation of reasonable cost-containment initiatives. At the same time, courts have been willing to expand traditional liability principles to managed-care organizations, thus imposing some constraints on managed-care delivery. At this point, courts seem willing to defer to the market and have been quite reluctant to overturn managed-care initiatives based on public policy considerations, with several courts specifically deferring allegations that managed-care incentives violate public policy to the legislatures (see, e.g., *Ambroze and McClellan v. HMO of Pa.*, 604 A.2d 1053, 1056, footnote 6 (Pa. Super. 1992)) and other courts rejecting challenges to the essence of managed-care cost-containment initiatives. If these trends continue over a range of cases, the decisions will have important implications for a number of health policy and health-care delivery considerations.

First, the willingness to uphold cost constraints will implicitly limit physician autonomy. Indeed, the courts' unwillingness to reject UM on public policy grounds indicates a willingness to accept limitations on physician autonomy. Even if courts defer to physicians on malpractice standards, that courts have upheld economic credentialing, staff selection and retention restrictions, and utilization management decisions suggests that physicians will not retain their prior dominance over the allocation of health-care resources. The implication of the litigated cases is that the courts' traditional deference to the treating physician is not likely to be sustained.[24]

In part, this is a very ironic result. Previous commentators have argued that the courts supported the prior model of physician dominance by deferring to physicians in developing standards of care for medical malpractice cases (Kapp 1985; Havighurst 1995). Physicians, who have long resented medical liability doctrine, may now attempt to hold onto it as the best mechanism for retaining their autonomy in health-care delivery. By upholding contractual restrictions and other limitations, however, courts may simply be doing what they have done in previous eras—deferring to the market winners. In the past, the market winners were the physicians; now MCOs are the market winners, and courts are deferring to them.

What has changed over the past decade or so to cause the courts' shift from protecting physician dominance to reinforcing managed care's dominance? At this point, the answer is somewhat speculative because of the limited number of cases. One potential explanation for this shift is that courts are responding to the changes in the underlying health-care environment, in this case to the expansion of managed care. As the nature of health care has changed, especially the prominence of cost-containment goals, it is perhaps not surprising that courts have begun to incorporate those goals in resolving managed-care litigation.[25] Though the trend toward contract is neither unlimited nor uniform, it represents a potentially significant departure from the cases reviewed by Professors Hall and Havighurst, among others, where courts showed greater willingness to scrutinize and overturn contracts based on contractual ambiguity (Mooney 1995).

This raises three questions. First, as a normative proposition, should MCOs be immune from negligence actions based on reasonable cost-containment programs? Second, as an empirical proposition, will the imposition of liability unduly constrain the development of cost-containment programs? Third, in developing legal doctrine, will courts shift from the dominant tort law paradigm to contract law in resolving disputes? From a conceptual perspective, there is no reason why MCOs should be automatically absolved (as a matter of legal doctrine) of the adverse consequences of their economic decisions. Numerous commentators have argued in favor of enterprise liability that would further solidify the MCOs' control of medical care, at the expense of being held accountable for adverse medical outcomes (see, e.g., Havighurst 1997; Abraham and Weiler 1994; Sage, Hastings, and Berenson 1994). The question is whether the standard should continue to be based in tort or should shift to contract law. Despite the urging of several commentators (Havighurst 1995; Morreim 1995), courts have only hinted at the possibility of shifting to contract-based determinations (see, e.g., *Dukes v. U.S. Healthcare,* 57 F.3d 350 (3rd Cir. 1995)).

To be sure, the potential for liability places a constraint on the extent of cost containment. But in doing so, the courts would simply be playing their traditional role in setting limits and in monitoring private economic relations. By imposing general negligence standards, the courts would not be impeding cost-containment initiatives but would be requiring plans to weigh the costs and benefits of doing so, given potential adverse medical outcomes. The question is, what standard should MCOs be held to in implementing cost-containment programs? While a full discussion of this issue is beyond the scope of this chapter, there is no reason why MCOs should be prevented from arguing that the proper negligence standard should incorporate cost-based decisions. In essence, juries should be able to decide whether the MCO has balanced the benefits of preserving assets for the patient population relative to the harm incurred by the individual patient, as in any other industry (Schwartz and Komesar 1978).

Second, these cases have implications for legislators and regulators. As a general proposition, courts have been hesitant in holding MCOs accountable for cost-containment initiatives that have an adverse effect on individual patients. This may reflect uncertainty on the desirability of imposing liability at the expense of cost containment, may reflect deference to the underlying policy judgments made by the market and by the legislatures, or may indicate a willingness to weigh the needs of the patient population above that of the individual patient (Morreim 1995). From a policy perspective, the result is functionally equivalent: at the present time accountability resides with the legislatures, not the courts.

In bioethics cases, courts have been willing to make decisions that many argued were best left to the legislature, even when legislators were unable or unwilling to do so. In the areas discussed earlier, courts are sending the message that restrictions on managed-care innovations should be made by the legislatures, not by the courts. Whether the courts will eventually set broad parameters (i.e., this far and no further), particularly in liability, remains to be seen. In any event, public dissatisfaction will need to be remedied by the legislatures; the courts do not seem inclined to interfere with the market. For physicians, the implications are that courts will no longer reflexively defer to physician autonomy. Physicians, too, will need legislative support for that.

Third, as Hadorn (1992) and Hall and Anderson (1992) have noted, courts are likely to insist on proper procedural mechanisms to protect individual patients. The unresolved issue is whether courts will eventually defer to procedures established by MCOs, as Hall and Anderson (1992) have proposed, or whether courts will essentially impose such stringent procedural requirements that are tantamount to limitations on implementing stringent cost-containment initiatives (see, e.g., *Grijalva v. Shalala*, 152 F.3d 1115 (9th Cir. 1998), cert. granted, judgment vacated, 1999 WL 66707 (U.S. May 3, 1999)). Courts may well seek a middle ground, but such a compromise position has yet to be articulated.

Fourth, physicians should consider whether their medical practice autonomy would be better served by supporting the current ERISA law, which essentially impedes the states' ability to monitor MCOs (see, e.g., Mariner 1996), or by supporting changes to ERISA that would enhance state regulatory mechanisms. This, essentially, is a question of whether physicians believe that they have more to gain by eliminating ERISA preemption than they have to lose by being subject to state legislative oversight.

For several reasons, this analysis should be considered preliminary. First, managed-care litigation is still in its early phase, making it premature to assess clear trends. In particular, the hard cases likely to emerge, such as adverse consequences from pharmaceutical restrictions or limitations on costly technologies, have not yet reached the courts. Second, the analysis relies more on leading cases than it does on a representative analysis of cases. Third, there is considerable state-to-state variation in legal doctrine that must be considered before consistent trends can be identified. This chapter has, of necessity, provided a broad scope rather than a carefully nuanced approach. Fourth, the line between deference to the legislature and expanding common law is a delicate one.

Conclusion

The tort system, through litigation between private parties, serves a valuable function in ordering private relations between unequal parties in a new and changing environment. In health-care litigation, courts have been reluctant participants in setting the parameters of acceptable cost-containment innovations for two interconnected reasons. First, courts have broadly interpreted ERISA preemption to block adequate consideration of the challenges to certain managed-care initiatives. Second, courts have not adequately understood the nature of the underlying transactions and changes in health-care delivery, making it difficult to develop doctrine that balances legitimate cost-containment policy goals with the courts' traditional concern for protecting individual access to goods and services.

Right now, the tension between managed-care decisions favoring patient populations at the expense of individual access to services is being implicitly resolved in favor of patient populations. Courts might not be conscious of the implications of case-by-case challenges to cost-containment strategies, yet the policy implications are that courts are deferring to the market to order these relationships. Whether the courts will reconsider current doctrinal development must await the accretion of cases expected to emerge during the next few years.

A Final Note

In a closely watched decision, *Pegram v. Herdrich* (530 U.S. (2000)), the Supreme Court confirmed some of the trends described in this chapter and may have changed others. First, the Court held that patients covered by an ERISA plan cannot sue to challenge an MCO's use of financial incentives to limit health-care services. Ruling that public policy has encouraged the use of financial incentives to reduce health-care costs, the Court essentially said that concerns about managed care should be resolved by the legislative branch, not by the courts. This opinion removes any doubt as to the judicial acceptance of managed care's cost-containment programs.

Second, the Court cast doubt on the ability of ERISA-covered patients to sue under a breach of fiduciary duty theory. While this part of the opinion is not entirely clear, the Court's approach suggests that it does not view managed care's hybrid financial-benefit decision making as amenable to a fiduciary duty challenge.

Third, the Court reaffirmed its opinion in *Travelers,* suggesting, at least for now, that the quality-quantity distinction as articulated by the lower federal courts is an acceptable development. The Court did not decide how to distinguish between quality and quantity for purposes of ERISA preemption.

Fourth, the overall tone of the opinion is very favorable to managed care. The Court is clearly deferring to Congress and to the market to set the terms of health-care delivery. Although it is possible to read the opinion as opening managed care to state-based litigation, the overall tenor of the opinion indicates that the complexities of managed care are matters best resolved through the political process.

NOTES

This chapter was written in the spring of 1997 and was subsequently edited in March 1999.

1. In social science research, a random sample of cases would be the preferable methodology. That methodology has rarely been used in legal research, although the research that forms the basis of this article will, in part, pursue a random sample. In litigation, however, not all cases are created equal. Some cases—by virtue of the reputation of the particular court or judge, because it may set precedent, because it is the sub-

ject of extensive scholarly commentary, or because it is cited by other courts—become more important than other cases. Thus, legal scholars focus on prominent cases, as will I in this chapter.

2. *Black's Law Dictionary,* 6th ed. (St. Paul, Minn.: West, 1990).

3. Morreim (1989) argues that courts should bifurcate the standard of care into a technical component (maintained by all physicians) and a resources component that would allow different standards of care as a function of available resources. In a managed-care environment, this would allow MCOs to defend cost-containment challenges based on allocating plan resources to various uses, such as preventive care. Havighurst (1995) argues that the standard of care should be determined contractually, essentially allowing providers to bargain with patients over the level of care to be provided. Abraham and Weiler (1994), along with others, argue that courts should shift medical liability from physicians to the enterprise providing the care, such as an IPA or other MCO. This standard, known as enterprise liability, would provide the enterprise with greater incentives for monitoring the quality of care.

4. Testimony of Meredith Miller, Deputy Assistant Secretary, Pension and Welfare Benefits Administration, before the Committee on Labor and Human Resources, U.S. Senate, March 24, 1998.

5. See, e.g., recent cases denying damages for wrongful denials of care, including *Turner v. Fallon Community Health Plan, Inc.,* 127 F.3d 196 (1st Cir. 1997), and *Andrews-Clarke v. Travelers Insurance. Co.,* 1997 WL 677932 (D.Mass. 1997).

6. *Pacificare of Oklahoma v. Burrage,* 59 F.3d 151 (10th Cir. 1995); *Dukes v. U.S. Healthcare* 57 F.3d 350 (3rd Cir. 1995).

7. For example, a complaint was filed on March 18, 1997, in *Castillo v. Humana, Inc.,* No. 97-1917, Fla.Cir.Ct., alleging that agreements between primary care providers and the defendant HMO that could limit referrals to specialists were not disclosed to subscribers. Plaintiffs allege that these undisclosed provisions constitute a conflict of interest and fraudulent inducement to enroll based on a level of care unlikely to be provided.

8. Although the independent contractor doctrine (insulating institutions from liability for the acts of independent contractors) appears to be eroding, some courts have not held IPAs vicariously liable for the actions of independent physicians (see, e.g., *Raglin v. HMO Illinois, Inc.,* 595 N.E.2d 153 (Ill.App.Ct. 1992)).

9. See, e.g., *Wickline v. State of California,* 239 Cal.Rptr. 810 (Cal.Ct.App. 1986), and *Sarchette v. Blue Shield of California,* 223 Cal.Rptr. 76 (Cal. 1987).

10. See, e.g., *Bush v. Dake,* No. 86–25767, Mich. Cir. Ct., Saginaw County, April 27, 1989, and *Berel v. HCA Health Services of Texas, Inc.,* 881 S.W.2d 21 (Tex.App. 1994). In *Bush v. Dake,* the court held that it is an issue of fact as to whether UM incentives contribute to medical liability. The case settled before trial.

11. See also *Tolton v. American Biodyne, Inc.,* 48 F.3d 937 (6th Cir. 1995), and *Corcoran v. United Healthcare, Inc.,* 965 F.2d 1321 (5th Cir. 1992).

12. *Lancaster v. Kaiser Foundation Health Plan,* 958 F.Supp. 1137 (E.D.Va. 1997), and *McClellan v. HMO of Pa.,* 604 A.2d 1053, 1056, footnote 6 (Pa. Super. 1992). However, the widely noted case of *Fox v. Health Net of California,* No. 219692 (Cal. Super. Ct. 1993), resulted in a substantial settlement following a $90 million jury award for Health Net's refusal to pay for a bone marrow transplant. Fox challenged the role of the defendant's financial motivations in the clinical decision.

13. I am indebted to my colleague Edward Goldman, JD, for this observation.

14. See, e.g., *Self v. Children's Associated Medical Group,* Cal.Super.Ct, No. 695870, 1998, where a jury awarded damages to a physician who was fired in violation of a California statute for providing too many tests and spending too much time with patients.

15. Indeed, in *Moore v. The Regents of the University of California,* 793 P.2d 479 (Cal. 1990), the California Supreme Court held that "a reasonable patient would want to know whether a physician has an economic interest that might affect the physician's professional judgment," but it did not challenge the underlying transaction.

16. Cited in the Bureau of National Affairs' *Health Law Reporter* 6:1235–36 (August 7, 1997). See also *Ehlmann v. Kaiser Foundation Health Plan,* 1998 U.S. Dist. LEXIS 13326 (N.D.Tex. 1998) for a similar result.

17. Such extraneous language is known as dicta. Although dicta cannot be cited as part of the legal holding in the case, it provides insight into the court's thinking and how it might approach similar cases.

18. See, e.g., *Crocco v. Xerox Corp.,* 956 F.Supp. 129 (D.Conn. 1997), 137 F.3d 125 (2d Cir. 1998), and *Murphy v. Board of Medical Examiners of the State of Arizona,* 949 P.2d 530 (Ariz.App. 1997).

19. Antitrust cases can be private or public law cases. In private law cases, individuals or groups can bring an antitrust case to protect private interests. In a public law context, the state or federal government brings the action to protect competition

20. Department of Justice and Federal Trade Commission, "Statements of Antitrust Enforcement Policy in Health Care," Washington, D.C., August 1996.

21. For a similar analysis, see Rosenblatt, Law, and Rosenbaum 1997.

22. See also, *New Jersey Psychological Association v. MCC Behavioral Care, Inc.,* 1997 U.S. Dist. LEXIS 16338 (D.N.J. 1997).

23. The Hall et al. (1996) regression analysis attributes this result to being in federal court rather than to ERISA. But for a critique of these results, see Sage 1998.

24. An exception to this is *Muse v. Charter Hospital of Winston-Salem, Inc.,* 452 S.E. 2d 589 (Ct.App.N.C. 1995), a case that did not involve an independent utilization management firm. The court deferred to physician autonomy where the plaintiff was discharged when his insurance coverage expired. The court held that the treating physician's recommendation of a continued hospital stay should have been honored, leaving open the question of who pays for the continued hospitalization, given current economic incentives. Arguably, this result is more consistent with cases decided before the expansion of managed care. See, e.g., *Van Vactor v. Blue Cross Association,* 365 N.E.2d 638 (Ill.App. 1977).

25. In *Doe v. SEPTA,* 72 F.3d 1133 (3rd Cir 1995), and *Creason v. State Department of Health Services,* 957 P.2d 1323 (Cal. 1998), the courts explicitly made this trade-off. See also Morreim 1995.

REFERENCES

Abraham, K., and P. Weiler. 1994. "Enterprise Liability and the Choice of the Responsible Enterprise." *American Journal of Law and Medicine* 20 (1–2): 29–36.

Anderson, G. F. 1992. "Courts and Health Policy: Strengths and Limitations." *Health Affairs* 11:95–110.

Blum, J. D. 1996. "The Evolution of Physician Credentialing into Managed Care Selective Contracting." *American Journal of Law and Medicine* 22 (2–3): 173–203.

Blumstein, J. F. 1994. "Health Care Reform and Competing Visions of Medical Care: Antitrust and State Provider Cooperation Legislation." *Cornell Law Review* 79:1459–1506.

Eddy, D. M. 1996. "Benefit Language: Criteria That Will Improve Quality While Reducing Costs." *Journal of the American Medical Association* 275:650–57.

Ferguson, J. H., M. Dubinsky, and P. J. Kirsch. 1993. "Court-Ordered Reimbursement for Unproven Medical Technology." *Journal of the American Medical Association* 269:2116–21.

Furrow, B. R. 1997. "Managed Care Organizations and Patient Injury: Rethinking Liability." *Georgia Law Review* 31:419–509.

Greaney, T. L. 1994. "Managed Competition, Integrated Delivery Systems, and Antitrust." *Cornell Law Review* 79:1407–1545.

———. 1997. "Night Landings on an Aircraft Carrier: Hospital Mergers and Antitrust Law." *American Journal of Law and Medicine* 23:191–220.

Hadorn, D. C. 1992. "Emerging Parallels in the American Health Care and Legal-Judicial Systems." *American Journal of Law and Medicine* 18:73–96.

Hall, M. A. 1988. "Institutional Control of Physician Behavior: Legal Barriers to Health Care Cost Containment." *University of Pennsylvania Law Review* 137:431–536.

———. 1989. "The Malpractice Standard under Health Care Cost Containment." *Law, Medicine and Health Care* 17:347–55.

———. 1997. *Making Medical Spending Decisions: The Law, Ethics, and Economics of Rationing Mechanisms.* New York: Oxford University Press.

Hall, M. A., and G. F. Anderson. 1992. "Health Insurers' Assessment of Medical Necessity," *University of Pennsylvania Law Review* 140:1637–1712.

Hall, M. A., T. R. Smith, M. Naughton, and A. Ebbers. 1996. "Judicial Protection of Managed Care Consumers: An Empirical Study." *Seton Hall Law Review* 26:1055–2069.

Havighurst, C. C. 1995. *Health Care Choices: Private Contract as Instruments of Health Care Reform.* Washington, D.C.: AEI Press.

———. 1997. "Making Health Plans Accountable for the Quality of Care." *Georgia Law Review* 31:587–648.

Jacobson, P. D. 1989. "Medical Malpractice and the Tort System." *Journal of the American Medical Association* 262:2230–37.

Jacobson, P. D., and S. Pomfret. 1998. "Form, Function, and Managed Care Torts: Achieving Fairness and Equity in ERISA Jurisprudence." *Houston Law Review* 35:985–1078.

Jacobson, P. D., and C. J. Rosenquist. 1988. "The Introduction of Low Osmolar Contrast Agents in Radiology: Medical, Economic, Legal and Public Policy Issues." *Journal of the American Medical Association* 260:1586–92.

Kapp, M. B. 1985. "Medicine and Law: A Symbiotic Relationship?" *American Journal of Medicine* 78:903–7.

Mariner, W. K. 1996. "Liability for Managed Care Decisions: ERISA and the Uneven Playing Field." *American Journal of Public Health* 86:863–69.

Mooney, R. J. 1995. "The New Conceptualism in Contract Law." *Oregon Law Review* 74:1131–1206.

Morreim, E. H. 1989. "Stratified Scarcity: Redefining the Standard of Care." *Law, Medicine and Health Care* 17:356–67.

————. 1995. "Moral Justice and Legal Justice in Managed Care: The Ascent of Contributive Justice." *Journal of Law, Medicine and Ethics* 23:247–65.

————. 1997. "Medicine Meets Resource Limits: Restructuring the Legal Standard of Care." *University of Pittsburgh Law Review* 59:1–95.

————. 1998. "Benefits Decisions in ERISA Plans: Diminishing Deference to Fiduciaries and an Emerging Problem for Provider-Sponsored Organizations." *Tennessee Law Review* 65:511–53.

Rosenberg, G. N. 1991. *The Hollow Hope: Can Courts Bring about Social Change?* Chicago: University of Chicago Press.

Rosenblatt, R., S. Law, and S. Rosenbaum. 1997. *Law and the American Health Care System.* Westbury, N.Y.: Foundation Press.

Sage, W. M. 1998. "Judicial Opinions Involving Health Insurance Coverage: Trompe L'Oeil or Window on the World." *Indiana Law Review* 31:49–73.

Sage, W. M., K. E. Hastings, and R. A. Berenson. 1994. "Enterprise Liability for Medical Malpractice and Health Care Quality Improvement." *American Journal of Law and Medicine* 20 (1–2): 1–28.

Schwartz, W. B., and N. K. Komesar. 1978. "Doctors, Damages and Deterrence." *New England Journal of Medicine* 298:1282–89.

Appendix A: Glossary of Terms and Acronyms

AAHP. The American Association of Health Plans is the principal national trade association representing HMOs, PPOs, and other managed-care organizations. It represents approximately one thousand health plans that serve over 140 million Americans nationwide.

AWP. Any willing provider laws have been enacted in approximately twenty-three states. They require managed-care plans to accept any provider who is willing to accept the terms and conditions of participation in the plan.

CISN. Community integrated service networks, licensed by the insurance commissioner to provide health services to fifty thousand or fewer enrollees, must maintain a minimum network of at least $1 million.

COBRA. The Consolidated Omnibus Budget Reconciliation Act of 1985 allows for the continuation of employee health coverage benefits in certain circumstances.

ERISA. The Employee Retirement Income Security Act was enacted in 1974 to provide for national uniform administration of employee pension and health plans through federal legislation and to promote the growth of these private plans by freeing them from state laws.

Gag clauses. When contained in managed-care contracts with physicians, these clauses seek to restrict physicians from discussing all appropriate medical options with their patients. Most states now ban such clauses.

HCFA. Health Care Financing Administration

Health Maintenance Organization Act of 1973. This act encouraged the growth of managed care by offering incentives.

HEDIS. The Health Plan and Employer Data and Information Set are performance measures developed by NCQA.

HIPAA. The Health Insurance Portability and Accountability Act of 1996 requires insurance portability from job to job.

HMO. Health maintenance organization

IPA. Independent practice association

IDS. Integrated delivery system

MCO. Managed care organization

NAIC. The National Association of Insurance Commissioners is a private regulatory program.

NCQA. The National Committee for Quality Assurance is a private accreditation program.

PHO. Physician hospital organization

PSO. Provider sponsored organization

RBPG. Risk-bearing provider groups take a variety of forms, including IDSs, IPAs, PHOs, and PSOs.

Appendix B: Managed Care On-line Resources

Compiled by Raj Gupta and Jeanne Kin

Government

Health Care Financing Administration
http://www.hcfa.gov
Statistics and published data concerning Medicaid and Medicare programs

Associations

American Association of Health Plans
http://www.aahp.org/AAHP/index.cfm
Information and statistics published by the major national trade association for managed-care organizations

Association for Health Services Research
http://www.ahsr.org
Provides useful links for researchers

National Committee for Quality Assurance (NCQA)
http://www.ncqa.org/Pages/Main/index.htm
Nonprofit accrediting body for managed-care organizations; information on health plan quality standards and accreditation

Health Plan Employer Data and Information Set (HEDIS)
http://www.ncqa.org/pages/programs/HEDIS/index..htm
Links to information concerning HEDIS

Physicians and Health-Care Professionals

American College of Managed Care Medicine
http://www.acmcm.org
Nonprofit society offering educational programs for physicians and other health-care professionals

American College of Physicians–American Society of Internal Medicine
Managed Care Resource Center
http://www.acponline.org/mgdcare/index.htm
Managed-care resources for physicians provided through the nation's largest medical specialty society

American Board of Managed Care Medicine
http://www.abmcm.org
Offers certification program in Managed Care Medicine

National Association of Managed Care Physicians
http://www.namcp.com
Nonprofit association serving the interests and needs of physicians working in managed care; promotes physician-directed managed health care.

Physicians for a National Health Program
http://www.pnhp.org
Organization of physicians advocating a universal, comprehensive single-payer national health system

Management and Policies

Advisors for Health Care
http://www.managedhealth.com
Health-care consulting firm; provides links to key industry sites

Aon Healthcare Alliance
http://www.aonalliance.com
Peer discussion forum sponsored by health-care consulting firm for health-care risk management, managed care, and HR consulting professionals to exchange ideas and solutions

The Institute for Health and Productivity Management
http://www.ihpm.org
Nonprofit institute focusing on relationships between employee health and workplace productivity

The Institute for Managed Care (Michigan State University)
http://www.healthteam.msu.edu/imc
Interdisciplinary center promoting education and study in the effective delivery of managed care; links for educators, legislators, administrators, health professionals, and students

Kaiser Family Foundation
http://www.KFF.org
Philanthropy focused on health-care issues; useful links for health policy analysts

Managed Care Information Center
http://themcic.com
Provides access to publications, on-line databases, and managed-care industry news

Patient/Consumer

Families USA Foundation
http://www.familiesusa.org
"The Voice for Healthcare Consumers"

"Patient's Guide to Managed Care"
http://www.panpha.org/HMOGuide.htm
Guide to Medicare Managed Care, produced by the Pennsylvania Association of Non-Profit Homes for the Aging (PANPHA)

National Organization of Physicians Who Care
http://www.pwc.org
Anti-HMO advocacy group news and views

HMO/PPO Medical Insurance Breakdown
"Consumer Protection Healthcare Handbook"
http://www.DrAnonymous.com
Anti-HMO site for patients, run by an anonymous practicing physician

Publications
The American Journal of Managed Care
http://www.ajmc.com
Home page of journal publishing peer-reviewed literature on health care outcomes; information for health-care professionals and health services researchers

Managed Care
http://www.managedcaremag.com
Information for managed-care executives and physicians on health insurance and delivery issues

Contributors

The American Association of Health Plans (AAHP) is the principal national trade association representing HMOs, PPOs, and other managed-care organizations. AAHP represents approximately one thousand health plans that serve over 140 million Americans nationwide.

Gail B. Agrawal, J.D., M.P.H., is professor of law at the University of North Carolina at Chapel Hill, School of Law.

George Anders is senior special writer with the *Wall Street Journal* and the author of the book *Health Against Wealth.*

James F. Ball is a senior advisor for Health Care Initiatives at General Motors Corporation.

John E. Billi, M.D., is the associate dean for Clinical Affairs at the University of Michigan Medical School.

Bruce E. Bradley is the director of Managed Care Plans, Health Care Initiatives at General Motors Corporation.

Troyen A. Brennan, M.D., J.D., M.P.H., is the president of Brigham and Women's Physician Hospital Organization and is a professor of medicine at Harvard Medical School.

Bruce Bullen is the commissioner for the Massachusetts Division of Medical Assistance and is the chairman of the National Association of State Medicaid Directors.

Clifton R. Cleaveland, M.D., M.A.C.P., is a clinical professor of medicine in the University of Tennessee's Clinical Education Department, Chattanooga, and is a practicing general internist.

Keith J. Crocker, Ph.D., is the Waldo O. Hildebrand Professor of Risk Management and Insurance and a professor of business economics and public policy in the University of Michigan Business School.

James C. Cubbin is the executive director of Health Care Initiatives at General Motors Corporation.

Cathy L. Hurwit has widespread experience in the formulation of health policy and in the drafting of health-care legislation. She has worked as the legislative/deputy director of Citizen Action from 1982 to 1987 and from 1990 to 1997. In addition, she has served as a legislative affairs specialist for the American Federation of State, County, and Municipal Employees (AFSCME) and as the legislative director for Rep. Ed Markey of Massachusetts. She is currently the chief of staff for Rep. Jan Schakowsky of Illinois.

Peter D. Jacobson, J.D., M.P.H., is an associate professor in the Department of Health Management and Policy at the University of Michigan's School of Public Health.

Jeanne M. Kin is a staff associate in medical school administration at The University of Michigan Medical School.

John R. Moran, Ph.D., is a research fellow in the Department of Health Management and Policy at the University of Michigan's School of Public Health. He holds a postdoctoral fellowship from the Robert Wood Johnson Foundation.

Alice A. Noble, J.D., M.P.H., is a professor in the Department of Health Policy and Management at the Harvard School of Public Health.

Margaret E. O'Kane is the president of the National Commission for Quality Assurance in Washington, D.C.

Deborah Salerno, Ph.D., is a project associate with the University of Michigan Medical School administration.

Frances Wallace, M.A., is the director of the Health Benefit Plans Division of the Michigan Insurance Bureau, Lansing.

Index

AAHP. *See* American Association of Health Plans

AAMC. *See* Association of American Medical Colleges

Academic medical centers, 9–11, 15, 83–102

Access to care, 9, 16, 24, 36–39, 46, 53n. 16, 78, 96, 105, 137, 146, 148, 157

ACOG. *See* American College of Obstetricians and Gynecologists

ACP. *See* American College of Physicians

Aetna Inc., 29n

AFL-CIO, 122, 133

Agency for Health Care Policy and Research (AHCPR), 41, 122, 133

Agrawal, Gail B., 3–17, 205

AHCPR. *See* Agency for Health Care Policy and Research

American Association of Health Plans (AAHP), 13–14, 24, 67, 80, 153–63, 199, 201, 205

American Association of Retired Persons (AARP), 122, 133

American College of Obstetricians and Gynecologists (ACOG), 36

American College of Physicians (ACP), 9, 63–64, 66–67, 202

Anders, George, 7–8, 12, 15, 18–28, 205

Anti-trust laws, 5, 16n. 7, 90, 183–85, 188, 195n. 19

Any willing provider (AWP) laws, 34–35, 37, 68, 126, 161, 199

Association of American Medical Colleges (AAMC), 85–86, 93

AWP. *See* Any willing provider laws

Balanced Budget Act of 1997, 40, 47–48, 89, 154, 169

Balanced Budget Refinement Act (BBRA), 89

Ball, James F., 120–34, 205

Barents Business Model, 162

Barents Group, 14, 153–63

BBRA. *See* Balanced Budget Refinement Act

Billi, John E., 9–10, 15, 83–102, 205

Blue Cross Blue Shield, 64, 108, 167

Bradley, Bruce E., 12, 13, 120–34, 205

Brennan, Troy A., 8, 12, 15, 29–57, 205

Budget Conciliation Act for 1998, 69

Budget Reconciliation Act of 1995, 98

Bullen, Bruce, 12–13, 135–41, 205

Bush, George, 18, 29n

Bush, George W., 21, 53n. 16

CAHPS. *See* Consumer Assessment of Health Plans Study

California Cooperative HEDIS Reporting Initiative (CCHRI), 150

California Medical Association, 73

Capitation, 23, 68–69, 91, 128, 176, 182

Centers for Disease Control (CDC), 122

Chafee, Sen. Lincoln (R-RI), 53n. 16

Chronically ill patients, 12, 15

Cigna's provider network, 42–43

CISN. *See* Community integrated service networks

Cleaveland, Clifton R., 9, 15, 61–71, 205

Clinton, Bill, 20

Clinton Health Care Reform, 68

COBRA. *See* Consolidated Omnibus Budget Reconciliation Act of 1985

Committee on Performance Measurement (CPM), 149

207